D0110672

Breast Cancer Survivors' Club

A Nurse's Experience

Breast Cancer Survivors' Club

A Nurse's Experience

Lillie Shockney

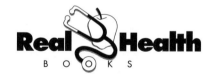

Loveland, Colorado

Breast Cancer Survivors' Club:
A Nurse's Experience

Copyright 1999 by Lillie Shockney
All rights reserved

Written by Lillie Shockney

Reproduction in any manner, in whole or in part
in English or any other language, including usage of electronic,
mechanical, information storage or retrieval systems, or
any systems developed in the future without the express
written permission from the publisher and author, except by a reviewer, under the Fair
Usage Doctrine, is strictly prohibited.
Any unauthorized use of any of the contents of this book
may result in civil penalties or criminal prosecution.
This copyright is registered with the U.S. Copyright Office,
Washington, D.C., and is protected under copyright law,
and internationally with all member countries of U.S./foreign copyright treaties.

PRINTING HISTORY
1996, 1997, 1999, 2000

For information contact:
Real Health Books
243 E. 4th St.
Loveland, Colorado 80537

PRINTED IN THE UNITED STATES OF AMERICA
10 9 8 7 6 5 4 3

Dedication

This book is dedicated to:

My husband, Al, for showing me that his love for me is eternal.

My daughter, Laura, for sharing with me the
wisdom and humor that a loving child can provide
in a crisis situation.

My parents, who provided me with their continued love
and support and reaffirmed my belief that
"once a parent, always a parent."

The late John Cross, for being my guardian angel.

My surgeon, Charlie Yeo, for having the surgical skills
and professional compassion to
help me become a breast cancer survivor.

Foreword

Thank God for Lillie Shockney, a true champion dedicated to the cause of cancer patients! I promise that you will both laugh and cry at the same time while reading Lillie's story. She has unselfishly given us a very intimate insight into her fight and victory against breast cancer. This story is not about Lillie, though; it is entirely about helping you, the reader, learn how to cope successfully with a cancer diagnosis, whether you are the patient, a family member or friend of the patient, or a health-care provider. Lillie documents how a positive outlook, lots of laughter, proper medical care, and prayer and faith in God brought her safely through treatment to become a new member of the "Survivors' Club."

It has been said that eternal vigilance is the price of freedom. Early detection saved Lillie's life—twice. Her story re-emphasizes to us all the importance of constant vigilance in the fight against this cancer and other cancers. It certainly has inspired me to make sure my own mother is doing breast self-exams and getting yearly mammograms. Other vital issues to be addressed in the new millennium include national standards for breast cancer care, elimination of unnecessary delays from time of diagnosis to time of surgery, continued public education, and research into true preventive measures—in addition, of course, to early detection efforts.

Lillie has a genuine servant's heart for helping other cancer victims, and she certainly will be involved at the forefront of these issues. I'm blessed to know her, and after reading her story, you will be, too.

Aaron Tabor, M.D.
Medical Director of Physicians Laboratories

Contents

Chapter 1

I guess it is best that we don't know what our future holds in store for us, because if we did, we'd probably convince ourselves that we'd rather not go through the experience—even if the end result is sometimes a positive one. I once read on a bumper sticker the definition of an experience:

*"An experience is what you get
when you don't get what you want."*

Those of us who have had breast cancer, still have breast cancer, or love someone with such a diagnosis are among those who have had "an experience."

I've had the unique opportunity to experience breast cancer from three different perspectives: as a teenager who watched the impact that a diagnosis of breast cancer had on someone I loved and feared losing; as a registered nurse who cared for women treated for this disease; and as a woman who became a mastectomy patient. This book is about these three experiences and how they affected and continue to affect my life and the life of my family. I will be very candid with you, because I feel that it's important for you to be given an opportunity to gain a sense of how this disease may affect you.

If you are a woman who has been diagnosed with breast cancer or fear contracting breast cancer in the future, I hope you find the information about my experience helpful emotionally, physically, and spiritually. If you are a nurse or other health care professional involved in the care and treatment of women with breast cancer, I hope you gain a sense of what it's like to be on the receiving end of such care. After all, with one in eight women being diagnosed with breast cancer, you could one day be in my shoes (or, rather, my bra).

I also provide resource information for breast cancer patients, families, and friends who are in need of access to medical information, emotional support, or other services.

This is my story.

From the time I was born I have had a variety of experiences with ill health. From the moment my mother brought me home from the hospital as a newborn I had boils all over my body from a staph infection. In three months, it had advanced into pneumonia. By the age of three I began to experience other health emergencies, like the time I found out what would happen if a toddler dropped a glass gallon jug on cement and then stepped on it.

And so the experiences continued—measles, mumps, chicken pox, a broken hand, sprained ankles, a broken nose, chronic tonsillitis, ear infections, lacerations, puncture wounds—the list goes on and on. You name it, and this young elementary school girl experienced it. The irony of it is that I always looked healthy. My brother, three years my senior, was the one who looked as if his health were borderline throughout most of his childhood. But with the exception of a few predictable childhood illnesses, he maintained excellent health despite his appearance.

Born and reared on a dairy farm in Maryland, I had lots of opportunities for experiences with accidental mishaps—which I guess is why my parents always made sure I had a tetanus shot every spring. I used to get really mad at them about that shot. You see, my brother got to go to camp every summer, and as part of the camp regulations he had to get a tetanus shot. I, on the other hand, didn't get to go to camp, but they made me get a tetanus shot anyway. Now, as an adult, I can see that they were using good judgment and saving themselves a repeat trip to the doctor's office, nearly an hour away from our farm, because before the summer was out I would have needed a tetanus shot anyway.

This is probably the reason they never let me go to camp—I was an accident looking for a place to happen. Every year I'd ask, "Can I go to camp with Robert?" Every year the answer was, "You are not old enough to go to camp." One year when I asked my annual question, the response was different. They replied, "Camp? Why, you are too old to go to camp." (Gee, I guess my opportunity to "experience" summer camp would have been the winter of my eleventh year of age.)

As you might surmise, whenever I, the adult, am mad at my folks, I usually throw in a zinger such as, "And by the way, you never let me go to camp, either!" In that way, they know I still think I should have had the experience of injuring myself in a fun location instead of having my medical mishaps occur only on the farm.

Whether I felt the need for medical expertise so I would know how to take care of myself, or whether my compassion led me to want to take care of others—what drove me toward a career in nursing is still a mystery to me. I'd like to believe that it was (and still is) the compassionate side of me, but part of my brain may have been reaching back into my childhood wanting to make absolutely sure that all those trips to the doctor's office (and all those tetanus and penicillin shots) were truly necessary.

Even through high school I struggled with health problems, especially respiratory problems, and I seemed forever to be on some type of antibiotic. But I nevertheless looked healthy. I had just started my teenage years when a couple moved to a home not far from our farm, and the wife of the couple took a liking to both me and my mom. Though she was at least ten years older than my mother, "Miss Bertha" (as I chose to call her) had the spirit of a child. I was basically a loner in school, partly because I was known as a bookworm and partly because I didn't live near enough to other children to play with. Our farm was nine miles from the next town and more than one mile from the nearest family with children.

So despite the fact that Miss Bertha was old enough to be my mother (or possibly even my grandmother), she became a best friend to me. She enjoyed inviting me over and practicing cheerleading routines with me. She also taught me how to sail a sailboat she had. It was just a small sailboat, a thirteen-foot sloop, but it was wonderful. When we sailed, all the pressures of school, teenage life, and farm work were far from my mind. I don't know what kind of pressures this woman had because she never discussed them with me. But the moment the wind made a whooshing sound and snapped the mainsail and the jib with a thrust of air, the look on her face was one of serenity. We rarely talked about the problems that either one of us was having; our time together was spent forgetting those troubles.

Miss Bertha's world took on a different perspective, though, after she went to see her doctor about an open sore on her breast that did not heal. Unfortunately, twenty years ago, women were not as well-versed on the warning signs of breast cancer. Billboards saying "Go get a mammogram once a year for the rest of your life" were not displayed along the highways as they are today. So although Miss Bertha was a well-educated woman with a master's degree in psychology, she did not realize that the bloody drainage from her nipple, a sore that would not heal, and a palpable mass in her breast meant major trouble for her and those who loved her.

When Miss Bertha was given the diagnosis of breast cancer, she was dumbfounded and perplexed. My mother was very concerned for her, and I was afraid I would lose her. Most people didn't talk about breast cancer then. You could say she had cancer, but it was taboo to say it was "breast" cancer. Thank heavens things are different now, at least in most social circles.

Miss Bertha had a total radical mastectomy, and most of the time remained cheerful and her old upbeat self. About a month after her surgery, she asked me to look at her scar to make sure it was healing okay, because a small spot was still weeping a tiny amount of drainage each day. I remember her saying to me that she felt comfortable with my seeing it because I was going to be a nurse and would know if anything was wrong. What I really think she was seeking that day was not a medical opinion about her incision, but acceptance of her appearance. I had never seen someone's scar after a mastectomy and did my best to maintain a flat affect and not show shock.

But I was shocked. Her cancer was advanced enough that the

surgeon had felt the need to remove the breast, muscle, lymph nodes in the arm and axillary area, and a few ribs, which meant that skin had to be grafted to her chest wall to close the wound. I could literally see her heart beating. The sight was quite scary to me.

Despite my inner feelings and my youth, I mustered the courage to say that I thought it "looked very good and was healing as anticipated." She was so pleased to hear me say those words that she hugged me very close, despite the fact that her chest was, I'm sure, still very tender. Having someone who loved her accept her as she was must have been very important to her at that time.

Although Miss Bertha was married, she seemed not to be blessed with a loving husband to help her endure such a medical crisis, and she had to rely on others for emotional and spiritual support. Crises such as these, I find, either bring a married couple closer or drive them farther apart. I suppose for her, marriage was somewhat of an "experience." But what is that old saying? "Love may be blind, but the neighbors ain't" fits many marriages. Perhaps Miss Bertha and her spouse were happy with one another; they just didn't seem to demonstrate it in the public eye.

Miss Bertha got a breast prosthesis a few months after her surgery and seemed back to her old self again. One day while she waited for me outside in her bathing suit, ready to walk to the beach at the foot of their property, I went to use the bathroom in her house. Lying on the bathroom counter was an object that looked like a thick jellyfish. I picked it up and discovered that it must have been her prosthesis! It certainly didn't look like a breast, nor, to me, feel like a breast, and I never asked her any questions about it. I was convinced, though, that the inventor of the device lacked an understanding of what a breast prosthesis should look and feel like. I thought that someday, if I had the opportunity to influence the designers of the future, I would give them my opinion of what a prosthesis should be like.

Miss Bertha had a friend who'd received bilateral mastectomies for cancer, and her friend visited as often as time would allow, even though she lived out of state. She was a neighbor to Miss Bertha's sister in New York and a very likable lady. I had the opportunity to meet her on several occasions and found her to be much like Miss Bertha—able to get on with her life despite the experiences life had dealt her. Miss Bertha acted differently when she was with her friend. It is hard to explain, but I could see it on their faces and hear it in their voices. They took great pleasure in telling funny stories about their individual experiences with breast cancer.

I'd like to share two of the stories that stand out in my memory. I remember them from more than twenty years ago. Miss Bertha's friend told us that after she'd had her second mastectomy she realized that she could be whatever bra size she wanted to be. She bought an inflatable bra, and for a time was very happy with it. It was lightweight and allowed her to do the gymnastic routines she enjoyed without any fuss. Because she had been very buxom before her surgery, she usually had her bra inflated to the max. One day she was going out of town to visit a family member some distance away, and, as always, was wearing her inflatable bra. She didn't realize that was an unwise practice when traveling by air.

There are lots of signs in an airplane that instruct you about what to do and what not to do. Signs tell you where the exits are and signs tell you not to smoke. There are even live demos and videos showing what to do in the event of a crash. But there are no signs that warn, "If you are wearing an inflatable bra, we strongly recommend that you deflate it before take-off or the pressure in the cabin will cause it to explode." Yes, you guessed it. She said they were airborne about fifteen minutes. She was engaged in conversation with the man in the seat next to her when all of a sudden—POW POW—her bra exploded. Despite this shocking occurrence, she made believe nothing happened. She took the sweater from her lap, slipped it around her shoulders, and buttoned it. When the opportunity presented itself, she scurried to the restroom and used tissues to fill what the atmospheric pressure had deflated. She merely chalked it up to an experience in the life of a breast cancer survivor. Good for her!

The second story that I want to share with you is one that

happened to Miss Bertha just a few months after her mastectomy. She was having a lot of trouble getting her arm's full range of motion back, so she decided to take up golf. Because she'd found the exercise of walking her fingers up the walls a little silly, she wanted an exercise that would not make her feel she was wasting her time. (Of course, I know of some people who find hitting a little white ball around a field of green grass equally silly, but she was not one of those people.)

She decided that she'd need a golfing instructor to teach her the proper techniques, so she signed up for lessons. The instructor, unaware of why Miss Bertha was taking up golf, assumed, as anyone would, that she was interested in the sport. However, her progress as a golfer disappointed her instructor, and he constantly told her to "swing all the way through." One day, about four weeks into her private lessons, she did swing all the way through as he wanted, and out fell her breast prosthesis onto the grass. (This was before bras were made with pockets to hold a prosthesis in place.) Miss Bertha looked at the object lying on the ground as if it had landed there from outer space. She couldn't bring herself to pick it up, because she didn't want her instructor to know that it was hers and, worst of all, to know what it was.

But the instructor took the initiative and picked it up. As he handed it to her he asked, "Why didn't you tell me that you've had a mastectomy? I need to teach you different techniques to get your full swing working for you!" How marvelous that this man took the steps necessary to make her feel perfectly comfortable with herself and with him. I never met this golf instructor, nor do I know his name, but I instantly admired him when I heard this story.

I mentioned that Miss Bertha acted differently when she and her friend were together. It wasn't that they acted weird—although Miss Bertha was known for doing funny things in strange places, like the time we were in New York City together and she decided we should skip down Fifth Avenue. The difference was that a special connection existed between the two of them spiritually and emotionally whenever they were in each other's presence. I've seen this kind of special connection between babies twelve to eighteen months old who see one another from their strollers in the aisle of a department store. I saw it once when two children with Down's syndrome met by chance on a street corner and hugged, even though they did not know each other. They clearly recognized that they had something very special in common.

As a breast cancer survivor, I now know what the special connection shared by Miss Bertha and her friend feels like. It is truly special and only for club members. To be a club member, you must have had breast cancer. It is obviously an elite club—not one for which you find membership forms in the back of a high-society magazine.

Neither Miss Bertha nor her friend are alive today. Their time as survivors of breast cancer was not meant to be eternal, but they truly made the most of their lives and touched the hearts of many who knew them.

About ten years after Miss Bertha was originally diagnosed and treated for her breast cancer, she had a recurrence in the form of bone cancer. It was then she told me that she had always wanted to have a child of her own but had not been blessed with the opportunity. She had been pregnant once, but had miscarried at five months.

She felt as if I were the child she had never had. She admitted to me that when we were in public, if someone asked whether I was her daughter, she answered "yes." She was glad to have me as her "borrowed" daughter and thankful that I wasn't her real daughter, because she would have felt very distressed if her having gotten breast cancer increased my risk.

How strange that even though Miss Bertha and I were not tied by blood, I eventually became a member of this elite club anyway. And now I must deal with the guilt and fear that my genes may pass this defiant disease on to my own daughter.

Chapter 2

My three years at Easton Memorial Hospital as a student nurse gave me ample time and opportunity to meet and provide nursing care to other "club" members who were diagnosed long before I was. The first experience I can recall having with a mastectomy patient occurred during my nursing rotation in the recovery room. It was common practice in the late sixties and early seventies for a patient to go into surgery not knowing whether she was about to get just a biopsy or receive a mastectomy. Patients were asked to sign consent forms that said, in essence, a breast biopsy was going to be performed and if the frozen section pathology results showed it was cancerous, then, while the patient was still under anesthesia, the mastectomy would be performed as well. Of course, if the biopsy was negative, no further surgery was needed.

From the viewpoint of the people scheduling the operating room, gathering the necessary surgical supplies, and arranging for other things needed in connection with a possible second surgery, it was all a matter of paperwork and stocking of shelves. But for the patient, it was fear of the unknown, literally. Going under the knife and not knowing until you awakened whether you had both breasts had to be a living nightmare.

I recall the first breast cancer patient I took care of in the recovery room. Her breast biopsy had been immediately followed by a total radical mastectomy. She awakened with a look of absolute terror on her face, and as I checked her blood pressure, she grabbed my hand and asked in a frightened voice, "Tell me, is it there? Is it gone? I don't want it to be gone. Please tell me that it isn't gone." My eyes connected with hers in a way that branded the image of her frightened face in my mind to this day. My silence told her the answer that she didn't want to hear. Her sobbing was like the cry of an injured animal trapped in a dark cavern. All I could think to say was, "I'm sorry." Sorry for her and, I guess, sorry for me. Sorry that her worst fears had been realized and sorry that I was the one to bear the bad news, even though I never actually confirmed for her that she'd had a mastectomy, or that the same agonizing day an additionally awful treatment for her advanced breast cancer was to follow. We cried.

Of course, other patients awakened with that same horrified look but were given good news. "Yes, your breast is still there. Your doctor will be in shortly to talk with you." Receiving confirmation that "it" was still there so elated each of these women that she felt no post-surgical pain upon hearing this good news. Instead, each reaction was one of euphoric laughter and happiness, as if I had told her that while she was under anesthesia her lottery ticket had just won her ten million dollars.

This analogy raises an interesting point. What is the value of a breast? Some women pay a great deal of money and go through considerable pain to have their breasts made bigger. Some who have lost a breast to cancer have undergone extensive and often risky surgery (such as a tram flap procedure) to have a breast recreated from other parts of their own flesh to "replace" the one surgically removed. Still others have desired no surgery to replace that which was stolen from them by this dreaded disease. Is that because a breast has no value? Or because the woman values it so much that a substitute or imitation is considered worthless—her lost breast cannot be replaced no matter how much money is spent or how much pain she is willing to endure?

I suppose the latter must be true because many women opt to have a lumpectomy rather than a mastectomy even though their doctors tell them that their risk of recurrence is greater. Some have refused surgical intervention at all because the cost of losing a breast is more than they could bear. These are the women who often sacrifice their lives to avoid, as they see it, being "dismembered."

I recall reading in *Dr. Susan Love's Breast Book* that in many cultures, breasts have a deep, often mythical significance for women. They are the external badge of womanhood. Although the uterus is the center of reproduction, it is invisible; it does not identify us to the world as female. When we see an androgynous-looking person, we instinctively glance at the chest to determine the individual's gender.

Sexual attractiveness is often correlated with the presence of breasts. "The bigger the better" is represented in erotic magazines and by skimpy swimsuits. Breasts have become a visible and outward symbol of femininity and sexuality. Yet you won't find women showing off their femininity by walking through grocery aisles naked from the waste up. To demonstrate such a physical display of their womanhood is not socially acceptable in western civilization (and thank heavens not, in my opinion). But a few women I've seen have come pretty darn close to showing it all!

This "let's see them—no you can't" attitude has added to society's confusion about how to deal with the topic of breast disease. Though the club is growing, we still have a long way to go before people feel comfortable discussing cancers that affect sensitive subject areas such as breasts and testicles. Perhaps the next generation, the one my child is part of, will deal with this issue differently. That generation is exposed to sexually explicit information at a sweet young age because of our need to prepare them for the pitfalls and risks of being sexually active (AIDS and STDs). As a result, children know more about sex in elementary school than I did when I got married at the age of twenty. Though I find that depressing and frightening, I do hope that the benefit will be the maturing of these children into young adults who are aware of the importance of good health and risk prevention, and who are open with one another in discussing their fears of certain illnesses such as breast cancer.

In 1988, I discovered a lump in my right breast. I was thirty-four years old and very frightened when I found it one morning in the shower. I contacted my doctor and he scheduled me for a mammogram the next day. I decided not to say anything to my coworkers. My reasons included my not knowing them very well, and because I was about to be promoted to a new job, I would be leaving the department anyway. But I also did not feel comfortable telling the fellows (all men) whom I worked with at the time that I might have a serious problem with my breast. So I took off during my lunch time, and knowing that the trip to the radiology building and back would probably take longer than an hour, I arranged to work late that evening.

When I arrived in the mammography suite I could feel the sweat running straight down my cleavage. My nerves were shot just thinking of what I might learn after the pictures were taken. That, I guess, was my first mistake. I expected to be told the answer immediately. If I had been willing to have the pictures taken at the hospital where I worked, a quick answer would have probably resulted, but I was in a strange place and answers were not forthcoming, as I had hoped.

First, the receptionist gave me a clipboard and asked me to fill out all the forms on it. These included not only the standard insurance papers but also a special diagram of a woman's breast that needed to be completed, too. The instructions said to check "yes" or "no" to a long series of medical questions. Then the papers instructed me to draw on the diagram where I felt the lump.

I checked "yes" to drainage from my nipple because since my child was born I had always retained milk. Even though I never breastfed, my left breast still contained milk—and she was in third grade at the time. (I used to joke with one of my friends that if I ever wanted to I could probably become a wet nurse!) In any case, I answered "yes" to this question. There was no space to write down that the drainage was milk, and there was no place to record that the milk was coming from the breast that felt fine and was "lump free." I then drew on the diagram where I felt the lump.

I was then taken into the X-ray room where mammograms were performed. The first time a woman has a mammogram is the one she remembers most vividly. When the technician picked up my left breast and placed it on the X-ray shelf, I felt as if she were scooping up a bag of marbles. Then the fun part came—the part where they try to see if it is really possible to take a large, round, dense mound of flesh and turn it into a quarter-inch thin pancake.

The answer to this question is yes, it hurts like hell before their smashing machine finishes converting you into breakfast food.

When the technician released the vise she tried the same routine on my right breast. This was the side I was worried about, and it hurt even worse while in the smashing machine than the first side did. Surely, this radiology device was invented by a man still very angry with his mother because she refused to breastfeed him, and as a teenager had been required to be home by 9:30 p.m. even on the weekends when he had a hot date.

The technician asked me to wait in the dressing room while the doctor looked at my pictures. But this is what I had been waiting for. I wanted to be with the doctor when she looked at my films. Nevertheless, I was told to wait. The first thing I did when I returned to the dressing room was to look at my breasts. I had the sudden irrational fear that when I picked up my hospital gown I would see two humongous flat pancakes hanging from my chest. Relieved, I put my gown back down and waited.

A few moments later the technician came and said, "You may get dressed now and go." Go? What did she mean, go? Certainly they wouldn't send me out the door without information about what the doctor saw? But they did. Despite my protests, despite my telling them that I was a nurse, they told me that my "doctor would send a report in the mail." Great. Now I'm also at the mercy of the United States Postal Service.

I returned to work feeling annoyed, but I rationalized that if the doctor had seen anything that was worrisome, surely she would have said something or at least asked me more questions about my lump. So I resolved to be satisfied and wait. At 5:30 p.m. my phone rang. It was the doctor from the radiology building. She was calling because she wanted more information. At least I had some privacy to talk because everyone from my immediate office area had gone for the day to begin a long holiday weekend. The doctor wanted to know how long the lump had been there, whether I had been having any bloody drainage, if there was any dimpling of my breast, and whether I had any history of breast cancer in my family.

I became very upset. I had filled out the papers, and except for not having had an opportunity to identify the kind of drainage, I had already answered all her questions. But the doctor said she wanted to make sure of the information because of what she saw on the mammogram. Oh no! What did she see? "I'm sorry, but I am not at liberty to discuss this with you. I will be having another radiologist look at the films on Monday and then we will be in touch with your doctor." What? You want me to wait to hear from my doctor?! I can't wait! Tell me now! She didn't though, and excused herself as she hung up the phone.

I started crying. A moment later when I looked up, there before me stood one of the men who worked in our department. He looked puzzled and concerned but definitely wasn't ready for what was about to come out of my mouth. When he quietly inquired whether I was all right and what was wrong, I responded by saying, "Oh, I don't know what I'm going to do. I think my breasts are going to fall off." This was obviously not the response he had anticipated. It was very unlike me to use such an expression. Moreover, he had no idea why I thought this strange phenomenon would happen to me. I then explained how I had spent my lunch hour, and he shared my concerns and anxieties of this unknown diagnosis. He helped me by trying to assist me in reaching my doctor, but the news only got worse. My doctor would be on vacation until the following Wednesday. His secretary said, "Oh gee, you just missed him. You nearly missed me, too, because I was just locking up to leave." I felt completely defeated, completely wasted.

That was an awful weekend for me. It had been planned as a very special one—the following day I was graduating from Johns Hopkins University, where I had finally completed my Master's degree in Administrative Science. My folks were coming over for the ceremony, and the day was planned to be a happy time. A time of celebration. But those plans were ruined. My husband and I decided that there was no reason to worry my folks with this health problem until we confirmed that it was a problem, so our concerns were kept secret. It was a long weekend, and an unpleasant and sleepless one.

On Wednesday of the following week I was successful in reaching my doctor and explaining to him the alarming call that I had received from the radiology doctor just hours after having left her department. He promptly called her and then called me back.

"Lillie, there is nothing to worry about. It's a blocked milk duct. Hot compresses and antibiotics will fix you right up."

A blocked milk duct? Then why did this female radiologist scare me to death? Come to find out she was a resident in training and quite new at reading mammograms. That was why she was having another doctor review them before a report was sent to my own doctor. All of that worrying for nothing. And to think that my graduation weekend had been ruined because of it. But now that I look back, I feel this was just a dress rehearsal for the real thing that would come five years later, when my breast really would "fall off."

Chapter 3

My experience in 1988 thinking that I had breast cancer caused me to reflect back to when I had cared for patients who were going through the same awful experience. The terrible waiting and not knowing, and always fearing the worst. In 1988, Al, my husband, was scared too. Scared for me. Scared for himself that he might lose me. We spent some time over that very long weekend talking about all of the "what ifs."

> Question: *What if it is cancer and I have to have a mastectomy, will you still love me?*
> Answer: *Of course.*
> Question: *What if I have to have chemotherapy and lose what is left of my hair? What will you think when you look at me?*
> Answer: *I will see you as I do now—my wife that I love very much.*

But God had been kind to me and spared me the experience of having to prove these hypotheses. And although it was just a dress rehearsal for a real experience at a later time, it gave me the chance to talk with the man I love so very much and to see what his reactions would be. Even though these were only words, they meant a lot to me.

Al and I decided not to tell my family or, for that matter, anyone, until we knew the verdict. Why worry people you love? They have enough of their own worries without my adding to them. So we told everyone that we had had a scare but that the scare was over. However, my folks were not pleased that they were not included from the start, and I promised them that if ever I had a scare again, I would let them know about it early on so they could lose as much sleep as the rest of us did. Never give up the opportunity to worry your parents. They expect it and will be angry with you if you don't. Somewhere there is an unwritten law that says if you have children you must assume full responsibility for their well-being, health, and level of happiness until one of you dies. The assumption is that the parents will die first; not because they are old and decrepit but because they worried themselves into an early grave. I share a belief in this unwritten law because we have a daughter of our own, and I can tell that I am going to worry about her and the various turns the path of life takes her on until I am pushing up daisies myself.

About a month or so after my mammogram I was able to stop thinking about my near experience with breast cancer and to stop focusing on my breasts and the status of their health. The lump went away just as my doctor said it would, and my life came back for the most part to its usual level of chaos. My respect for women who'd had the real experience crept up a few more points on my honor and respect scale.

I also started using more Ivory soap in the house too; purely as a reminder that its slogan that year was a good "take-home message," with TV commercials featuring young women who'd grown up in the country, wore very little makeup, and didn't need makeup because of their radiant beauty. Each woman on the commercial stood there looking lovely and very physically fit while her TV husband talked about how lovely his wife's skin was. The commercial closed with the slogan, "When you've got your health, you've got just about everything." Though I didn't think that washing my breasts each day in the shower with Ivory soap would become some new form of preventive medicine for breast cancer, I did think doing so would remind me of the importance and value of good health. We take for granted that which we have until we lose it.

My experience also inspired me to dig out a cross-stitched piece of work that I had made in high school and have it professionally framed. It depicts a well, and it reads, "When the well is dry we know the worth of water." So after that year I valued the appendages that hung from my chest all the more.

During the same month as my mammography scare I was promoted to the position of director of quality assurance, utilization, and risk management at Johns Hopkins Hospital, where I had been working for five years. It was a demanding job and required long hours and a lot of hard work. I took the responsibilities of this position very seriously. I loved the work. I guess I've always been a type A personality and got it from both my parents. My brother did as well. We're driven people—what they classify in the world of psychology as overachievers. The pace of this job and the demands of the political environment of the institution made it easy to forget about my scary experience the month before. Time passed quickly, and before I knew it, four years had sped by.

In April of 1992, at age thirty-eight, I began to have pain in my right breast. It was the same side where the blocked milk duct had caused pain before, so I wasn't too worried about it. I decided to use the warm compress treatment that I had used before, but this time it didn't work. So after three weeks of no relief, I decided to call the doctor. He ordered a mammogram.

This time the mammogram was done at the hospital where I work, and because of my position there, I know the majority of the physicians. Also because of my position, I am frequently treated like a VIP and am fortunate to get prompt service and medical care at a moment's notice. (Although I believe the care that Hopkins' physicians provide to patients overall is the best in the country, regardless of whether the patient has access to special contact people there.)

The mammogram was done by a mammography technician named Robin who was very compassionate and caring. She was in the right line of work, and I felt much at ease with her. I told her that I concluded, after having this second mammogram, that if ever the United States were to go to war again I knew the perfect weapon. The military should be provided portable mammography machines. Forget about the M16 rifles. Just let our side carry one of these metal vises. When they catch one of the enemy they can put his "three-piece set" in it and crunch down in the same way as with a woman's breast. Whatever military secrets the enemy might know would soon be secret no more, and the war would end quickly. (Al later said they could call it a gonadogram weapon.)

Robin completed the procedure, and when she asked me to wait in the booth for the films to be checked, I asked whether a particular radiologist I knew well was available to read the files with me. (I thought, there is no reason for me to wait for the verdict again. I'd prefer to discuss the results of these films right away. Besides, I was sure that the problem was minor and something similar to what I had experienced the first time in 1988.)

Luck was with me. The radiologist I asked for came into the room a few moments later. He said there was a cyst in the right breast—probably what was causing my pain. He paused a moment and then added that something visualized on the films taken of my left breast. There were "calcified" areas, and he wanted to get additional views of this breast taken. Calcified areas? Well, I decided not to worry about it until he gave me more information following the additional views.

Robin reappeared and took a few more pictures of my left side. About a half hour went by and the radiologist reappeared. He told me something was definitely there, but on enlarging the films the calcifications appeared to be spherical—which is usually a good sign. However, their pattern was in the shape of a horseshoe, and they seemed in the process of closing in to form a circle. Because of this he felt it wise to have me be seen by a breast surgeon for an opinion. And because he said that the possibility of this being breast cancer was extremely slim, I felt reassured. Thank heavens, I thought. A very gentle man, this radiologist stood tall and stoic, and he had a marvelous calming effect on nervous patients like me. So I left the radiology department without feeling concerned.

Over that weekend my gynecologist called me at home from the hospital and said he had received a copy of my mammogram, which he had ordered for me. He shared the radiologist's opinion and recommended that I go see a breast surgeon because of the "business" I was in.

I asked one of my staff people who she thought would be a good breast surgeon for me to see. I also looked through some of the quality assurance records that we keep on physicians as part of their credentialing process at the hospital. The surgeon she mentioned turned out to be an excellent choice based on the information available to me. No patient complaint data had been filed on him. His record showed virtually no infections or other post-op complications with his breast patients. The length of stay for his hospitalized patients was shorter than most stays—a plus in my book. (Being responsible for utilization management at the hospital causes me to look at patient care clinically and financially. Shorter lengths of stay are more medically optimal now than they used to be and usually better for the patient and her pocketbook.) This physician was considered to be an excellent surgeon by the operating nurses and floor nurses, and he was known to be compassionate, caring, and very thorough. I knew I would be in good hands. His name was Charles Yeo.

I was able to get an appointment with Dr. Yeo the same week, and he was as able and impressive in person as his paper credentials and the feedback from other health-care professionals had indicated he would be. He was also very handsome, another plus in my book. After being with him only a few moments, I thought how much he reminded me of my brother: straightforward, a precisionist, and highly charismatic.

The doctor examined my breasts and then showed me my mammography films, pointing out where the cyst was located on the right breast and where the calcified area occurred in the left breast. He believed, as the radiologist did, that there was probably nothing to worry about. He felt that the wise thing to do would be an open biopsy of the calcified area. At the same time he would perform a needle aspiration of the cyst in the right breast. I still felt very calm about the whole thing and left the exam room feeling that this procedure would be no big deal. Whatever the calcified area was, it was smart to remove it so it didn't create trouble for me later in life. The cyst's drainage via needle aspiration would be a piece of cake.

I contacted Dr. Yeo's secretary, who booked me for the minor surgery on June 2 at the Outpatient Center. When I got home that evening I told my husband the plans, and he, too, felt that it was nothing to worry about. I contacted my mother that evening and told her what was happening so she could spend three full weeks getting worried about it. And she did. So did my dad.

On June 2, 1992, I arrived at the Outpatient Center. Right away I was spotted by the medical director of ambulatory care, who was talking with a patient in the booth next to mine. Surprised to see me, he also checked on me several times during the day to make sure things were going as planned.

The full name of the procedure I had is "breast biopsy with needle localization," and I sum it up in one word—yuck. The beginning of the procedure involved placing my left breast in the mammography machine and once again smashing it down until it resembled a wad of dough waiting to be baked into a streusel. Then the fun part came.

A female radiologist arrived to insert a needle into my breast to serve as a guide for the surgeon in locating the calcified lesions. She explained that although breast tissue has very little feeling, I might feel a pinch. Using the X-ray as her guide to finding the spot in question, she jabbed the needle in me. A pinch? Maybe her breasts don't have much feeling, but mine certainly do! The pinch she thought I'd feel actually felt a lot more like a knife stabbing me. (I know of other women who have had this procedure, also without local anesthetic, who didn't complain of pain as I was experiencing.) The radiologist had some difficulty getting the needle in all the way because, as she explained, my breast tissue was very dense and further compressed by the mammography machine, yet compression was the only sure way to have the needle get to precisely the right spot.

I didn't know what to say or do. I was scared and trying not to show it. Picture it. My breast is being held captive in a vise with a ton of metal on it, and I have a needle hanging out of my body. I kept thinking about it, which was a mistake. Then I glanced down and watched her as she tried to get the needle farther into my breast. That did it. Looking. Watching the needle go in. I began imagining the sound a knife makes when you're cutting a potato in the kitchen. And...oh no. I started seeing spots before my eyes. The wall in front of me that had been a lovely shade of orchid became snow white. Then everything went white. I said, "I'm in trouble. I think I'm going to faint." That's what caused the chaos.

A blood pressure cuff was obtained and people hastened around me to get a chair. Ironically, I don't think I would have actually fallen. How could I? My breast was still in the vise! I couldn't have landed on the floor if I'd tried!

Smelling salts were stuck under my nose. I was apparently removed from the vise, placed in a cardiac lounge chair, and my feet propped up. After a few minutes the wall returned to its original shade of orchid and my face turned to red from embarrassment.

Statistically only about 2 percent of women having such a procedure actually fall in a faint. And even though they tell you "it could have happened to anybody," it didn't happen to just anybody. It happened to me. And I'm a nurse who has seen everything from gunshot wounds to the head to open trauma of the chest and even accidental limb amputations. All of that never bothered me. Of course, none of those patients were me. It's different if it happens to you, or someone you love, like your own child. The event is even more unpredictable because you don't know how you are going to react.

The radiologist finished this part of the procedure by injecting blue dye through the needle, which was still hanging out of me. The dye marked the area for the surgeon to excise. From the mammography room I was taken into a waiting area to be carted into the surgical suite. A cup was placed over the needle sticking out of my breast and taped in place to secure it.

Though I didn't like the procedure, I knew it was one of the more precise ways to pinpoint the abnormal area for the surgeon to excise the tissue that has been stained blue and to biopsy it.

My husband, Al, was able to be with me in this waiting area. That was reassuring. After a brief wait I was escorted into the surgery room. Once on the table, I knew that the show was ready to begin. Dr. Yeo came in already scrubbed and ready to go. He first drained the cyst in the right breast, which took only a minute. He then concentrated his efforts on the real job at hand. I was nervous and couldn't stop talking. The nurses in the room with me were very accommodating and allowed me to ramble on about the weather, vacation plans, and other such nonsense. Numerous times the surgeon injected me with a local anesthetic. My experience in the dentist's office has always been that I require a lot of that stuff before I'm genuinely numb. So was the case on this day. Periodically I would wince or say ouch, and I would get another shot in the breast area.

Dr. Yeo said he was surprised to find that I had severe cystic disease—he had to drain six cysts before he got to the area of the blue dye. The tissue mass that he removed was gray, and some good tissue was taken out as well for pathology to inspect. Finally I was stitched closed and the dressing applied. The procedure had taken about forty-five minutes but it felt like two hours.

About an hour later we were allowed to leave the hospital. Dr. Yeo told me as we left that he would be out of town for a few days and that when he returned he would call me with the results. He didn't want me to worry, though, and I didn't.

Al and I got home around 2:30 that afternoon and I felt pretty good. My mother had come over earlier because Laura, our daughter, had stayed home from school with a tummy ache. I suspected that it was from worrying about her mother, and it was. Laura doesn't even like hearing that someone has to have a shot, much less an operation, and if she is the patient, you'd better be prepared for an extra-awful day. She is truly terrified of needles and will faint at the sight of blood. Despite her having a very strong compassionate side, I doubt that she will end up in the health-care field unless she can be guaranteed that she won't have to do anything with blood, needles, and such.

My mother was glad to see me come home. She looked as I had imagined she would. Worried. Caring. Loving. Patient. She also had an expression on her face that confirmed for me that she had a whopper of a migraine headache. And why shouldn't she? Remember, I gave her three whole weeks to worry about today's events. She stayed until about six in the evening, then headed home to the farm, a two-hour drive away.

I stayed home from work for the next two days—not what I had originally planned. The local anesthetic wore off around 7:00 that evening and I felt as if someone had struck me in the chest with a baseball bat. I was also alarmed to see my incision. It wasn't what I had expected. But then, the degree of diseased breast tissue that the surgeon had removed was more than he had expected, too. The incision was about three-and-a-half inches long and it indented into my breast. When I raised my hand over my head it indented even deeper. I started to cry. Al comforted me and told me that I looked fine. That was the first time I realized how conscious I was about my breasts in relation to body image.

My secretary, Diane, stopped by after work the next day and brought me some papers that I wanted to work on at home over the weekend. Marge, one of my other staff members, had been by that morning to drop off some other work, which I had finished by the time Diane arrived. Diane is a special person to me. She's not just a great secretary (and we all know how hard that is to find) but also a very dear friend. Having her visit for a while and exchanging with her the completed work I'd done that morning helped me to feel productive that day. Her visit also reinforced in my mind how much she cared about me and loved me.

The next day, Saturday, Diane was planning to go into work. So I decided that instead of waiting until Dr. Yeo came back in town, I would have Diane check the results of my biopsy through the pathology database I had access to. Why wait to get good news? I was sure that the mass would be benign. Remember, these were calcified circles—not irregular in size. The procedure I'd undergone was merely preventive surgical care, I thought. Certainly this was not the beginning of an experience but the end of one. The pathology report wasn't ready, though, so I was unable to get a preview of this good news after all.

On Monday I went into work. My staff members were all supportive and empathetic. They too were anxious for me to get the good news so their anxieties could be relieved as well. But the report still wasn't ready.

On Tuesday afternoon I checked the database again. This time it said that the specimen had been sent to another pathologist for verification. Come on, people. Why was it taking so long to get this good news printed across my computer screen? When Tuesday evening came, many of my staff had been in and out of my office asking if I had the report results yet. Still the answer was no. Right before I got ready to leave, Diane, who stayed late with me, said, "The report is back. I checked it an hour ago. I wanted you to have privacy when you read it. I don't understand what it says."

I logged on and pulled up the report on my screen. It contained the usual medical terminology. It had words in it like "specimen," "tissue," and "cells," and then I read words that I was not prepared to read on any report that contained my name—"intraductal carcinoma." I read it over and over and still the same words appeared. The expression "out of the margins" also haunted me as I read more. I quickly logged off and asked Diane to go into the database with her password, thinking it would tell her something different. Not rational thinking on my part, but who thinks rationally when you are in shock? I had hoped that when she pulled my report up on the screen it would say "Ha, ha! Fooled you! That will teach you to look at your own report rather than wait for your doctor to call you on Wednesday." But that wasn't what it said. All the words looked the same as before. And the verdict was not what I had expected. It was cancer.

Diane was very upset but kept her cool. She said that the doctor had taken out the mass so there was nothing to worry about. I told her that I wasn't so sure, because the report said it was "out of the margins," which meant that some cancer cells were still left in the breast. Hurriedly she went to our other office down the hall and brought back a stack of our medical journals and reference books. While she was gone I copied the report down on paper and stared at the words before me. My head was swimming with images of awful things yet to come. Could this be a secondary metastasis from another primary site? Is it in both breasts? Is it in my lymph nodes? Am I going to die? What can I do to make all of this awful experience go away? I logged off the computer and stared at the dark blank screen as if I were looking at the Grim Reaper.

The textbooks were somewhat helpful because they refreshed my memory from my nursing school days. For the majority of patients diagnosed with breast cancer, it is not a death sentence. I wrote down information from these books, packed up my brief-case, and got ready to go home. Diane kissed me good-bye looking very worried—worried for her friend and trying to figure out how she could make all of this awfulness go away.

I walked down the corridors toward the exit where my car was parked. One of the hallways I passed, which I have walked by probably ten thousand times, was the corridor leading to the Oncology Center. I caught myself walking by it faster than usual to avoid the thought of perhaps having to enter those doors as a patient in the near future, perhaps fearing that as I walked by tonight the doors would spontaneously open and a great vacuum would suck me in. I made it to the car, and once I was alone I began to cry.

I turned the radio on very loud and pushed in a cassette tape of Natalie Cole's *Unforgettable* that I had recently purchased. Music has always been a great soother for me, and I have always found singing along with music to be very therapeutic. I sang and cried and sang some more. I knew that when I got home my husband would not be there. He had only recently begun helping out a friend of ours with a limousine service, who on occasion needed an extra driver. I knew Al had driven the limo to New York City that day to drop off some people who had rented it. He was not expected back until around 9:00. But I knew that Laura would be there, and I didn't want to upset her. I didn't want her to know that anything was wrong. So I pulled myself together, drove home, and parked the car in the driveway.

Laura could tell that I had been crying. She wanted to know what was wrong. I told her I'd had a bad day at work and not to worry about it. We had planned to go out for a "girls' dinner" since Daddy wasn't going to be home in time to eat with us. Although Laura was ready for dinner I told her that I couldn't go out. I didn't feel well and wanted to stay home, hoping that Al would get home sooner than planned. Her inquisitive mind persisted and she kept asking me if I was all right. I guess I wasn't very convincing that the problems reflected on my face were solely work-related. My brain was working on overdrive trying to figure out how to tell my husband, how to tell my parents, and how and when to tell my twelve-year-old child. My head ached, and I couldn't erase the vision of the computer screen with the words typed out so plain and cold: "carcinoma of the breast."

Chapter 4

Laura got herself ready for bed around 8:15 that evening, and I felt relieved. At least I had succeeded in sparing her a restless and nightmarish night. It gave me some comfort to know that she could rest unburdened by concerns about her mother's health.

The phone rang shortly after and I hoped desperately that it was my husband calling me from the limo car phone. My mother's voice asked, "Do you know anything yet?" I froze in place unable to speak. My silence gave her the answer to her question just as my silence had given the verdict to the very first mastectomy patient I had taken care of so many years before. I told her Al wasn't home yet and I'd rather call her back after he got home. My voice was soft in the hope that I would not awaken Laura, who had just gone to bed. Mom didn't want the conversation to end there, however. She wanted answers and asked me again about the pathology report. "Is it bad?"

I paused a few seconds, then answered with the one word "yes" and started to cry. I grabbed the portable phone and walked outside so Laura would not be disturbed. Now my mother was in shock. I felt thankful I didn't have to see her face at that exact moment. I knew how distressed she was, and direct eye contact at that moment would have been more than my heart could have handled. I told her I would call her back in twenty minutes and hung up the phone. Time was motionless. I wanted the clock to hasten forward so my husband would be home with me. At the same time I wanted the clock to go slowly so I could pull myself together and figure out how I was going to tell him that I had cancer. I also wanted to figure out something to tell my mother when I called her back that would make her feel better...something I could say that would let her know I would get through this—that we would get through this. The problem was that I wasn't sure I would get through this and survive this dreadful and potentially deadly development. All I knew was that I had breast cancer. I didn't know what stage of the disease I was in. I didn't know exactly what the treatment would be. I assumed that I would need a mastectomy but I wasn't absolutely sure of anything. I was able to collect myself and I called my mother back five or ten minutes later.

Her voice sounded strained as soon as she picked up the phone. I worried how she was going to deal with my telling her that I knew very little but that what I did know was bad. Having to say to her that I read my report and it said "breast cancer" must have been like pouring acid into her ears right through the phone. She was very upset that I would not be able to get any definitive answers tonight and would have to wait until I went to work in the morning and spoke to Dr. Yeo.

My mother told me that she loved me and I replied with the same. Somehow it sounded different—more tangible than I ever remembered hearing the words sound before. More intense. I told her that when Al got home I'd have him call her after I talked with him. She said okay and our conversation ended.

Only a few minutes later Al called on the car phone. I was very steady talking with him and tried not to project over the telephone lines that I was in major trouble. I didn't want him to get this news like my mother did, because he was traveling in a vehicle. I would be even more distressed if I said or did anything that jeopardized his safety behind the wheel. Our conversation was brief. He told me he would be home in about twenty minutes and began telling me about the day he'd had, but I really didn't hear much of what he said. I just clung to the words "I'll be home in twenty minutes." I wanted the time to once again race by so he could be home with me.

At 9:45 he walked through our kitchen door. He was very tired. He said he was hungry and began to go to the fridge. I stopped him and asked him to go downstairs to the basement with me. He looked perplexed by such an odd request and asked me why, but I just repeated my request to come downstairs. I didn't want our voices to be heard in Laura's bedroom. He followed me, and at the bottom of the staircase I stood in front of him and said, "I saw my path report. I have breast cancer." I was relieved to have the words out of my mouth. There, I've done it. He knows.

He looked at me in shock and said, "Well, that doesn't mean it's malignant, does it?"

I nodded yes. He grabbed me and squeezed me very tight. That moment will live in my memory for the rest of my life. I could feel his strength around me and knew that if it was possible to beat this, I could do it with his love. What he couldn't do for me was make it all go away. The whole thing was like a bad dream, a dream I wanted to wake up from but couldn't.

To complicate matters, Al had to return the limousine that night because the company needed it for a morning run. I didn't want him to go. He didn't want to leave either. First I thought that I could go with him, and then I remembered that Laura was in bed, so I stayed behind. He promised to hurry back, and when he left I felt a sense of panic. He said he'd be back within the hour. And he told me he loved me three times.

I felt frightened when I saw his taillights pull away. What was I to do with myself until he returned? Not just sit in a chair and wait. I had done enough of that already and it made me feel worse. I decided to empty the dishwasher, and upon completing that task I scrubbed out the shower in the master bathroom. If I'm going to die from cancer anytime soon I might as well have a clean house. I pictured people coming to my funeral and saying, "She sure went down fast. Gee, from diagnosis to death was only a week. But you know, her kitchen and bathroom looked and smelled really clean." I remember glancing at the bar of Ivory soap and decided to remove it from the soap dish. I replaced it with Coast, my previous favorite soap. The Ivory went into the trash.

Al returned within the hour, just as he'd promised. My link with life and survival walked through the door at 11:20 p.m. He told me that he didn't even remember driving down the beltway to Sandy's house, where he returned the limousine. Clearly his brain must have been on autopilot to have gotten him safely there and back to me. But the important thing was that he was back home with me, and all I desired at that moment was to feel his arms around me. As he and I stood in the kitchen holding each other tightly, I thought "protect me, make this awful thing go away." But I knew it was not possible for him to do. I also knew that he, too, felt frightened but was desperately trying not to show it. We both knew that this time it was not a dress rehearsal, as it had been four years ago. This was the real thing.

Al called my folks, as I had promised my mother he would. I don't know what they said to him, but I could hear him being remarkably steady on the phone. Amazingly steady. Confident. Confident that we would get through this experience. Confident that I would do well. Just hearing him tell my folks these words made me feel better. Of course he's right. Of course I will. "Please God," I thought, "make him dead right about this, because if he's dead wrong then I'm dead."

After he hung up, few words were spoken in our house. We went to bed around 12:30 a.m. We got undressed, turned off the lights, and held each other like two shipwrecked survivors riding out a furious storm. June 9, 1992, ended—the day I found out that I had been involuntarily drafted into the "club."

I rose early the next morning and went into work. My first mission was to call Dr. Yeo's office and get more information about my future, my life. His secretary answered the phone. She told me he was returning that day from having been out of town and would probably be in late. My heart sank. I explained to her that I had pulled up my path report on the computer and I needed to discuss the results with him right away. She said that their office had not yet received the report. I told her it was imperative that I talk with him because I knew that I had cancer. She told me she would put my file on the very top of his pile of work to review and would print off a copy of the path results for him to see. I thanked her and hung up. I must have stared at the phone for two or three minutes before I could get on with my day. I relayed to Diane, my secretary, what the status of my phone call was and she agreed to find me wherever I might be when the doctor called me back.

I tried to clear my head. I had work to do and needed to get on with it. Sitting by a phone waiting for it to ring would have turned me into a crazy person. So I went on with my meetings. The first meeting was with one of my bosses, Dr. Timothy Townsend. I had my usual long list of issues to discuss and make decisions about, and our meeting concluded without his having a clue that anything was wrong in my life. As I left Tim's office, Carole, his secretary and a long-time friend of mine, greeted me and handed me a long-stemmed rose with a card that read, "Thinking of you and hoping for the best." Carole was aware that I'd had a biopsy but unaware that I already knew the verdict. At least she was unaware until I made eye contact with her.

There is something about making eye contact that makes us more vulnerable at certain times in our lives. I stood before her silently and my tears began to flow down my face. I couldn't stop them. My silence continued. No words were needed. She promptly rushed over to me and hugged me. With that, Tim came out of his office. He asked whether I knew the results of my biopsy, and I nodded yes but could not bring myself to speak. After a moment of total quiet I said, "The biopsy was positive. I have breast cancer." Tim asked what Dr. Yeo had told me would be the next step. I floored him by saying that Dr. Yeo didn't know the results yet. I had looked them up on the computer myself.

Both Carole and Tim were very supportive. Carole felt bad that she had caused me to cry—I had arrived at their office looking fine and upon receiving a rose turned into a basket case. Heaven only knows what I would have done if she had handed me a lily. Tim walked me back to my office. Tim, by the way, is a pediatrician. Though the majority of his time then was spent as senior director of medical affairs, in my opinion, deep in his soul he is and always will be a physician. He has a warm personality, a genuinely caring mannerism, and a wonderful way with kids (and adults). He told me to call him as soon as I had heard from Dr. Yeo. He hugged me at my office door and departed.

Once I was back in my office, several of my staff members were anxious to know if I had my path results yet. A few asked Diane what the news was. She elected not to say and told them to ask me personally. (She told me she figured that this was my body and my business and that it wasn't her place to tell anyone about it. I admire her for that. I believe the thought of having to say those words might have been more than she could handle. She was very worried for me.) As folks came in and asked me, I mustered up the strength to tell them that the report was "positive." If a picture is worth a thousand words, I had the opportunity to get about six Kodak moments that morning. Everyone I spoke with was in shock. Everyone wanted to know the next step and hoped no further treatment was needed.

"He took out the lesion, so that should be all." That was the response from the majority. I knew in my heart that more treatment was to come. I could feel it within me. The report had said the cancer was "outside the margins," so there was still some left in there and it had to be disposed of somehow.

The day dragged along despite a fairly full schedule. At three in the afternoon Tim came by to check on me. To his "Any news?" I had to reply "No, I still haven't heard from the surgeon's office yet." I decided to call his office again and hoped I wouldn't be misrepresented as a pest. The thought went through my head that if I'm labeled as a pest maybe it will make the doctor mad and he'll want to take my arm off, too, along with my breast just for pestering his staff. (The adjacent arm was my left arm and I'm left-handed. It's the hand I use to hold the receiver of the phone.) Isn't it just awful the crazy things we think of when our brain is in one place and our body is in another?

Tracey, his secretary, again answered the phone. "I hate to bother you or Dr. Yeo, but do you know when he will be able to talk with me?" Tracey's response was not what I'd expected. "Gee, Mrs. Shockney, I'm really sorry. He was only briefly here and is gone right now. He'll be in touch with you in the morning."

The morning? Oh no. I didn't think that I would mentally make it until another eighteen hours had passed. She added, "He wants to discuss the path report with the pathologists and with Dr. Baker."

I felt like Dorothy in *The Wizard of Oz*. Remember when she had been through the awful experiences of being abducted by flying monkeys, having her dog taken away from her by the evil witch, was locked in a room with only minutes to live, and despite a myriad of obstacles managed to defeat the Wicked Witch of the West? The deal she had made with the Great Oz was that if she brought him the witch's broom he would get her home to Kansas. She brought him the broom and what did he say? "Come back tomorrow."

Well, I felt like running away to Kansas when his secretary said that I'd have to wait to hear from him "tomorrow." Tomorrow was forever to me. Can you imagine telling a woman in hard labor to "just keep panting until tomorrow"? Why, she'd punch your lights out! But I had no one to punch. I was too wasted to fight with anybody. So I tried to fantasize that maybe he could talk the pathologists into changing their minds and rewriting that path report. He could say, "Hey fellas, this lady is really nice. How about lightening up a little and rewording that report to read, "Great-looking breast tissue. Looks like it belongs to the body of a twenty-five-year-old."

The evening dragged on, as the day had. Al and I talked a great deal, and I told him I was 99 percent sure that my surgeon would be recommending a mastectomy. I was really scared about how Al would react to such a surgical procedure. I kept saying to him, "You don't know what this kind of scar will look like. The breast will be totally gone. Do you understand me? Gone. I will look awful. You might not want to look at me anymore."

But my husband remained just as steadfast that night as he had before, and—for that matter—as he had four years earlier when we'd gone through that awful dress rehearsal. "I want you well. I don't care what kind of surgery you need. I love you. We'll get through this. I love you." Then he'd hold me again and I'd cry. We each felt as if we were still in shock. I don't think either one of us could believe that any of this was happening to me, to us. I'm not sure what my parents were going through at this point, still lacking any definitive answers. Still not knowing what the future held for their child.

Among the meetings previously scheduled for the next day, June 11, was one with a financial consultant I had met once before at a seminar that the hospital had held for employees. I had planned to review with this gentleman the benefits and annuity arrangements that I had through my employer. A very personable man, Bud Leeb came in to my office at the appointed time and sat down, intending to review my financial profile so I could do as I'd intended—have him help me plan for my future and for my eventual retirement in twenty years. My retirement? Good heavens. Today was not a very good day for me to be looking at this kind of information. Today I didn't even know if I had a future or if I would live to see retirement. I didn't feel like talking about finances. What I needed was a lawyer to update my will. But Bud was very cheerful and pleasant, and I didn't want to ask him to leave and reschedule with me. He had traveled from his office downtown to meet with me, and I didn't want to impose on him again. So we proceeded with the meeting as planned.

As he began to talk with me he looked around my office and noticed the many cards and flowers that members of my staff had given me to lift my spirits. Bud asked, "Gee, is it your birthday?" I replied no, it wasn't. "Is it your anniversary or something?" I again answered no. He then said, "Well it must be a special occasion because you sure have lots of beautiful flowers and cards." And you guessed it—I disintegrated into tears. He was very alarmed, and he apologized for upsetting me and asked what was wrong. I told him I had just found out that I had breast cancer and was waiting to hear from my doctor at any time.

Bud then told me that his wife had been diagnosed with cancer many years before, and the doctor had given her a poor prognosis. She had a strong will to live and remained optimistic throughout her treatments and multiple abdominal surgeries. (She also obviously had a wonderful support system—her husband). He told me that he had no business troubling me today with numbers and for me to concentrate on my health and be optimistic. He gave me a hug and left my office swiftly. To think that he felt he was troubling me. For goodness sake, I was the one who had made the appointment with him!

About fifteen minutes later my secretary came to my door holding a basket of daisies with a card. It was from Bud. From that day forward he became a new friend and a member of my support system for the future.

At 11:15 a.m. the phone rang and Diane answered it. She promptly came to my door and nervously said that it was Dr. Yeo. She then closed my door to give me privacy. This was the call I had been waiting for. The little light blinking on my phone signaled the answer to my concerns about my life, my longevity, and my body. I picked up the phone and quickly grabbed a pen and paper.

"Mrs. Shockney, I hope you're sitting down because I'm afraid I have bad news." Bad news? Didn't he know that I already knew I had breast cancer? Unfortunately not. We discovered that the message he received had lost something in translation. He knew only that I wanted to talk with him as soon as possible about my biopsy results. He didn't know that I already knew what the path report said. He was stunned that I had been aware of the results for two days and now realized why I had placed two calls to his office.

He explained to me that when he had returned from his trip and reviewed the path report he wanted to talk directly with Dr. Silver, the pathologist, about the findings. He'd then met with Dr. Baker, known as an expert at the hospital in the field of breast cancer, for a second opinion about the best treatment options for me. Dr. Baker recommended a mastectomy. The other option was a lumpectomy with radiation, but Dr. Baker doubted that clean margins would be achievable at this point. Dr. Yeo suggested that I go home and discuss it with my husband—and I interrupted him. "What do you feel will give me the best chance of long-term survival? What would you tell me if I were your wife, your sister?"

His answer: "A mastectomy will give you the best long-term outcomes because you have multifocal disease."

So I said, "When do you want to do the surgery?"

He paused and said again, "Don't you want to discuss this with your husband?"

I explained that I had already and reminded him that I'd had two and a half days to think about this and was not surprised with his surgical recommendation.

I wrote down every word he said. Every word. I was proud of myself with how steady I was on the phone with him. But I also had the advantage of no required eye contact. I choked up only once and that's when we were discussing the date for surgery. He told me I was a strong woman and he was sorry I had had to deal with the knowledge of having cancer without knowing what the next step would be. I told him that I regretted looking up the information on the computer, but having access to this database was too tempting. Besides, I had felt so sure that the results would be benign, as the radiology and surgery physicians had predicted.

Dr. Yeo was very encouraging and I felt somewhat relieved to hear him recite the statistics on longevity, which sounded favorable to me. We discussed a date for surgery and I explained that my husband and I had planned a vacation the first week of July. I wondered if I should cancel it. "Definitely not. By all means get away for a few days. That way you'll be all rested up for surgery when you return."

We agreed on July 14. (He had suggested July 13 but I requested the following day because July 13 was the day I had married my first husband—now my ex-husband—and I had enough bad memories of that day without needing to add to them.) The doctor gave me the number of a clinical nurse specialist who would talk with me about the surgery, and I recorded her name and number. Our conversation ended at this point. My doctor was professional, charming, and—as always—thorough in providing me with all the information I requested of him. I elected to tell him that I was impressed with his thoroughness, the time he afforded me, and that it was physicians like him that made me proud to work at this hospital.

When I hung up, Diane must have seen the light go out on the phone because she opened the door to my office. On seeing Diane come in I started crying. She came over and put her arms around me. She asked what the doctor had said. "I'm scheduled for a mastectomy on July 14th." At that she cried even harder than she had before. I think she cried harder and longer than I did. Although I felt upset, I also felt relieved—relieved to know there was something that could rid me of this dreadful disease, optimistic that the outcome would not be a lovely bronze box covered with flowers, and confident that I was in the very best medical hands possible.

I called Al and told him what Dr. Yeo had told me, every word. Al was very positive. "A ninety-five to ninety-nine percent survival rate at ten years. Well, that sounds good to me. We're going to be okay, baby. I love you. It probably hasn't spread yet? That's a blessing. Even more to be relieved about. We'll get through this. We will. It will be okay. Do you want me to come and get you? Maybe you should be home. I just want to come and scoop you up and take you home with me and take care of you."

I thought how God had surely blessed me with a good husband. Al was truly a rock, and I needed him to be. I told him that I was going to continue my work schedule and not to worry. I'd call him before I left at the end of the day.

Diane and I went to lunch. We had only about twenty-five minutes before my next meeting. It didn't matter because neither one of us had much of an appetite. As I walked down the hall I was aware of an ache in my left breast. Purely psychosomatic pain. It hadn't ached all day until then.

My one o'clock meeting was with a group of my staff people. These are employees I spend a lot of time with, and I feel especially close to several of them. They had no idea yet that I had heard from the doctor. Only a few of them even knew at this point that my biopsy results were back. I didn't want to use this forum as the place to discuss my upcoming surgery. It was not an agenda item that I had planned to discuss in an open meeting. I wanted to do that in private. So I went into the rest room and tried to mentally collect myself. "You can do this," I said to myself. "Just push this problem out of your mind and get on with business. This is not the place to blurt out that you're getting your breast removed." So I took some deep breaths, composed myself, left the rest room, and entered the conference room door. Everyone was there so I took my seat and began. As I covered each planned agenda item on my list and discussed each topic, I caught my mind wandering, though only for a few seconds at a time. I was thinking, the people sitting here with me have no idea what I have just been told. They have no idea that I will be having my breast removed next month.

I felt a personal sense of pride that I was able to go on with "business as usual." It's part of my upbringing. To be a member of my family—an accepted member, that is—you'd better be productive. Definitely a German trait and one that survived many generations. I was glad that I'd been able to pull it off and felt hopeful that I'd be able to continue to conduct my work without this personal crisis affecting my productivity. That was important to me.

When I returned to my office I wrote notes to several members of my staff, people I am especially close to. I wrote that I had gotten the news from Dr. Yeo and that I was scheduled for a mastectomy. But it was hard to write it on paper. I looked at the words I had written and couldn't believe that all of this was really happening to me. As individuals came into my office after our group meeting and inquired, I directed them to their file folders where I routinely left them messages. It seemed odd to write this out rather than to simply tell them, but I had a fear of becoming hysterical if I had to say it too many times. Only a few special people did I have the nerve to tell face to face. Whether the individual read my words on paper and then returned to my office or heard the words stuttered from my lips, the response was the same. Tears. Shock. And without exception each person was stunned that I had been able to conduct the staff meeting just held without showing a hint of what I knew. This reinforced in me that I was a strong person. Stronger than perhaps I ever realized. But I knew that I was made from good stock and that what I had just done would have been expected, not a surprise at all to my folks.

I had other meetings that afternoon; one of them included Tim. I informed him of my news. His concerns for me were plainly visible on his face. He asked if it was all right if he told Chip of my situation and I said yes. Chip (Dr. Moses) was my other boss.

My mother called at work, which was rare. It is a long distance call and she calls only when there is a crisis. She left a message on my answering machine that Al had called her with the news from Dr. Yeo about my surgery. At the end of the day I called her back to let her know that I was okay, that somehow we'd get through this. I realized that I still needed to convince myself before I would be able to convince her. Her worries and fears could be heard in her voice. "Tell me what to do. I don't know what to do to help, to stop all of this," she said. There was nothing that she could do to stop it. It was what it was. This is where the meaning of the serenity prayer is oh so true.

God grant me the serenity to accept the things that I cannot change, the courage to change the things that I can, and the wisdom to know the difference.

These are wise words but sometimes very hard to follow. My mother knew she had no control over the fact that I had cancer. But despite her wisdom she struggled to figure out a way to gain control over it. This was the first time that my mother had not been the pillar of strength for our family. Our family had been through many other crises—a house fire, a barn fire, the devastating loss of all the crops one year, other serious illnesses, death of loved ones—and she had always been the strong one. But somehow this medical crisis engulfed her in a way that made it nearly impossible to deal with. And I worried about her. How could I shelter her from this pain? My intent was to find comfort from her, but for a while that would not be possible, because she needed the comfort as much if not more than I.

When I left work that day and reached my car, the tears began to flow like a river. Again I turned up the radio loudly, the music blaring the whole way home. My mind was no longer distracted with meetings and business calls and memos. My mind was totally focused on me. My life. My mind was full of unanswerable questions. I felt angry, too. Why me? What had I done to deserve this raw deal? Had I taken the wrong fork in the road somewhere and didn't know it?

The year before had been a very difficult year for me. After having suffered with many months of stress I had spiraled into an acute depression that caused me to seek professional help. Severely depressed, I'd been in an awful pit of doom and gloom. It had taken a lot of hard work and help from family, friends, and a good psychotherapist to pull me out of that pit. This was to be my year to celebrate life. To have a great summer. And what happens? I get told that I have cancer and need to have my boob taken off. Why? What had I done to deserve such a punishment? At least I felt like I was being punished.

I remembered when I was in elementary school and the boys would say, "I heard that if you play with yourself your 'thing' will fall off. Do you think that it's true?" Gee, I didn't know. I sure was glad I wasn't a boy, though. I used to think if a girl touched her nipples a lot, maybe they would fall off, too. I made sure never to do that. As I drove home that night, I thought about all kinds of irrational things, such as maybe as a child I had fiddled with my nipples while I was asleep and now I'm being punished by the booby demon.

I got home and felt exhausted. I don't think I could have felt any worse if someone had pulled me through a keyhole.

Chapter 5

It was hard for me to picture telling Laura that her mother had breast cancer and had to have her breast removed. I knew, though, that trying to protect her from the inevitable news was not the way to go. Laura was a smart twelve-year-old. She and I had always been close and she could read me like a book. She was already suspicious that something was being kept from her, and it was only a matter of time before she would overhear Al and me discussing it, or worse, hear it from someone else. I decided to tell her that night. It was consoling to me that it was summer and that she wasn't in the midst of classes. It would be hard enough for her to deal with this news without the additional burden of keeping up her grades. I decided to wait until late evening when I was changing my clothes, and I asked her to come in the bedroom and talk with me for awhile. She stretched across the bed in her favorite position and said, "So, Mom, what do you want to talk about?"

I didn't really know how to say it. Even though I had rehearsed how I would tell her and what words I would say, when I looked at her face my mind drew a blank.

"I can tell that something is the matter. There's been too much whispering around here," she said.

"Yes, there's been a lot of whispering, I guess. Remember when I came home the other night and you kept asking me what was the matter with me? Well, I didn't want to worry you then because I didn't have enough information. Enough facts. But since then I've gotten more information and I'm ready to talk with you about it."

She sat up on the bed and looked very concerned. "Laura, you know that I had some surgery done on my breast a week and a half ago. It was a special test to see if what was seen on my mammogram pictures was anything to worry about or not. Well, the test results are finished now. Lots of different doctors, very good doctors, have looked at them and have talked with me. The test consisted of taking some of the tissue out of my breast and looking at it under a microscope. When the doctors looked at it closely that way they saw cancer cells in it. So I will be having my breast taken off to get rid of the cancer that's there. The surgery is called a mastectomy, and I will be having this mastectomy surgery done in a few weeks."

Laura looked dumbfounded. She also looked confused. "How will the doctor take it off?" she asked.

I explained that I would be put to sleep and the doctor would make a cut across the top of my chest and underneath my breast and remove all of the breast as well as some tissue and lymph nodes under my arm.

Because Laura doesn't like to see blood, needles, or anything that implies pain, I anticipated her customary reaction. Usually she puts her hand up to her mouth and says, "Don't talk about it. I'll faint." But this time she didn't. Her curiosity was too high and she wanted to understand exactly what I was talking about.

Breasts have always been a special focal point for Laura. She worried throughout her tenth and eleventh years of life that she wouldn't have big breasts. It was clear that the amount of peer pressure she was getting at school was causing a major worry in her life. "What if they don't grow? I'll be a freak. None of the boys will like me. I want big boobs like you have. What if it skips a generation and I have boobs like Mommom? That would make me feel awful because everybody is growing big ones in school but me."

Heavens. The things we worry about in our youth. My grandmother had large breasts but my mother is a tiny woman (size two). I, however, have large breasts like my grandmother, so I could see why Laura would make the correlation that this special "big boob gene" might have skipped her generation.

The kids were so fixated on this issue that I wouldn't have been surprised to see it listed as a subject on her report card. "Laura Shockney—Boob class. Grade: D. Comments from instructor— needs improvement. Not progressing as expected."

As a matter of fact, Laura was fixated on her breasts at age three. She loved to play dress-up and enjoyed wearing my jewelry. My mother had even made her a little lab coat that she wore to make believe that she was "a nurse like Mommy." Over the winter months that year I had noticed that Laura's nipples were very red and she complained that her chest hurt. After about five days of her continuing to complain at night when I put her to bed, and her nipples being persistently red and inflamed, I called our pediatrician. He agreed to see her the following morning, so I took off from work the next day to take her for her appointment. I thought that maybe this was some kind of infection. Mastitis? I was familiar with mastitis, having lived on a dairy farm. I also had personally experienced it after Laura was born. I developed a breast abscess that subsequently progressed into mastitis, which was very painful. Now my poor baby, all of three years old, might have it. I felt awful for her.

She sat in the waiting room with me, holding my hand tightly. She didn't like Dr. Wolfe, her pediatrician. Though he was always very nice and I felt he was great with kids, she associated him with "needle shots" and would have been thrilled to never lay eyes on his face for the rest of her life. When our turn came we went into the exam room.

"Laura, your mommy says that your chest doesn't feel good. Let me see your chest," said Dr. Wolfe. Laura reluctantly lifted her shirt, but her face showed displeasure at having to be in his presence. He looked at her nipples closely and pressed around them to feel for lumps. He then repeated back to me the information I had given him over the telephone. "So you say she has been complaining when it's time to go to bed that her nipples hurt? And that's been going on for about five days?" I confirmed with a nod. "Well, I don't think it's mastitis. I don't think it's an infection at all, but I think it can be easily cured." Great, I thought. So what is it? He turned to Laura and asked, "Laura, have you been touching your chest, your boobies a lot?" I was stunned by such an inquiry. But not as shocked as I was with the response from my child. "Yes. I have been pulling on them to help make them grow so I can look like Mommy,"

If I'd had false teeth in my head, they would have clappered right out and onto the floor at this point. The doctor said, "Well, that's what I thought. It would be best if you didn't pull on them so hard. That's why your chest hurts at night. You eat lots of vegetables and they'll grow all by themselves." Then he turned to me and said, "Well, now we know the cause and the solution. By the way, your bill will be thirty-eight dollars."

What? Thirty-eight dollars to tell me that my child had been pulling on her nipples? Oh well, you can bet your bottom dollar that the next time Laura had anything other than a true medical condition like chicken pox or strep throat I quizzed her thoroughly before venturing back to the pediatrician. A lesson well-learned that day. So as you can see, breasts have been a priority item with my child for a long time.

I sat beside Laura on our bed and looked at her beautiful green eyes. She had the look of anxiety as well as an expression of inquisitiveness, because I had told her I was going to be losing part of my body to cancer. Her first question was, "Are you going to die?" I told her that I didn't think so. God was the only one who knew when any of us was going to die, but that I had no plans for doing so any time soon. I had excellent doctors and the cancer had been caught early, based on the information available so far.

Next, Laura asked me some surprising questions. "Will they let you bring your breast home with you from the hospital? After all, it is yours. They have no right to keep it." This was something I didn't expect to be asked. I explained that I would not be bringing it home with me because I had no need to keep it and that the doctors would be doing lots of tests on it to analyze the tissue in it. It kind of made me choke up a little when I pictured in my mind exactly how the pathology department did these tests. Slicing it up like a deli clerk who had been asked for three pounds of thinly sliced ham.

Then Laura asked me whether the doctor would take my right

breast and move it to the middle of my chest. Now that is an interesting image. Definitely not your average feminine figure. When I asked my daughter why she would think this, she said that she was afraid I would look funny with one breast on only one side and would probably lean to the right when I walked. I told her I would not be having the remaining breast relocated and would instead have an artificial breast to wear in my bra on the left side to replace the one the doctor removed.

I took her into the living room and showed her in the Sears catalog what the breast prosthesis looked like and what the mastectomy bras looked like. She was intrigued. She especially liked the idea of having a pocket in the bra to put the prosthesis in, and I told her the story about Miss Bertha losing her prosthesis on the tenth hole of the golf course because her bra didn't have a pocket.

Laura said, "Well, that pocket can be used for other things, too, Mom. When you go to the ATM bank machine you can put your money in the pocket and that way nobody could steal it." I thought, I'm not sure I'll send this idea into *Woman's Day* magazine as the helpful hint of the month, but it's definitely something to keep in mind for future reference.

I encouraged Laura to ask me questions as she thought of them and to let me know what worried her about this experience that our family was going through. I also told her, "Mommy would look different," but I didn't elaborate on that point. We would have many opportunities to talk more about all of this. I also told her that I felt very sad about having to have this surgery and there would be times that I would be crying. I told her to just give me a hug and kiss and let me cry. I needed to cry and that was good for me to get those feelings out of my system.

Laura went to bed shortly after our talk. When I kissed her goodnight she looked to me as she had when she was three. Tiny, fragile, and oh so special to me. I gave her a kiss on the cheek called a bumblebee kiss—like I used to do when she was very small—and she squeezed me tightly.

That night Al and I sat outside on the deck, and I recapped the conversation I'd had with Laura. He looked amazed as I told him the questions that were the real stumpers for me. We started to develop black humor that night, and I realized just how powerful laughter and especially black humor could be. We talked about what a conversation piece my breast would make sitting in a large jar on the mantlepiece above the fireplace. When our friends came over we could say, "Now here is Al's deer that he shot two years ago in the mountains, doesn't it have a magnificent rack? Over here is the fifty-inch bluefish he caught in the Chesapeake Bay last summer. And, oh yes, this is Lillie's left breast. Isn't it lovely?"

We talked a lot that night about how fixated society is on breasts. The bigger the better. I told him that recently one of the construction guys working near the hospital had whistled at me. I was sure that this worker was a boob man because I was wearing a cashmere sweater that particular day. I told Al, "Well, after the surgery, if that guy is out there and whistles at me again I'll yell over to him that now he's only half right!"

We joked about other things, too. "Gee, there has got to be an easier way to lose weight than this method. I guess I'll be leaving the hospital about five pounds lighter." Al got a big charge out of Laura's suggestion about where to hide the money that I'd withdraw from the ATM. Although it would definitely be a safe place to keep the money, I didn't know what the reaction would be when I needed to get it out to pay a bill. Can you picture me in the grocery store? The cashier would ring up the bill and I'd go rooting for my money. By the time I got the cash out of my bra, either the police would be there to arrest me for indecent exposure or the store would be empty because of people screaming and running for their lives.

Al was very sensitive, and very clever. He rarely offered the humorous quips himself. He let me do that. It was far better to have me be the jokester than for him to say something and catch me at a bad time when I might not find it so funny. He was happy to hear me tell these funny stories and knew that my doing so was good for me. And it was good for him. Laughter was like a special tonic. It lifted our spirits and kept us thinking in a positive way. It still does.

Chapter 6

I gave Al the unpleasant assignment of calling his family and telling them the bad news. His mother was very concerned and emotional about it because Al's older brother, Jack, had lost his wife to cancer of the colon and liver, and my mother-in-law feared I'd be the next daughter-in-law to go. Jack was very struck by the news, too. After his wife's death he had moved to a neighborhood not far from ours and routinely spent a lot of time with us. Just as he was piecing his life back together again, he was delivered news that sounded all too familiar to him, and he didn't want a repeat of his experience to happen to me or to his brother. Al's younger brother, Denny, just couldn't believe it. My age and the fact that I had never smoked or drank or done the usual and customary things that correlate to cancer left him perplexed.

I had several weeks before my surgery. I had asked for this extra time so I could get things organized at work prior to my surgery date. My job was a stressful and hectic one. A lot of tension was involved in dealing with issues that related to the quality of medical care, to potentially compensable medical and surgical events, and to problems for patients resulting from an insurance company's not covering the bills issued by the hospital and doctors. The job was very fast-paced, and in an institution the size of Johns Hopkins Hospital, a mammoth one. But I loved it and always gave 110 percent to my work there. (Remember, I'm a product of two overachievers.)

Because of my job, however, I was and still am blessed with access to the best medical care in the country. I feel bad for patients who have to travel blindly through today's healthcare system, having to figure out if they are receiving "good" care and trying to decipher where and how to get medical advice. (See the resource section in Appendix B, page 213, for more information on this issue.) It must be very hard and extremely nerve-wracking, particularly when the patient is in a life-threatening situation such as a diagnosis of cancer. Time is of the essence, and choosing the wrong doctor or treatment regimen can be potentially fatal for some individuals.

When I went to work on June 12, I was approached by other members of my staff about the status of my biopsy results. A lot of tears flowed over the next few days. Mine and the folks who worked for me. I did not want this medical crisis to disrupt my ability to be productive, and I wanted to get on with my daily activities. Each day I'd tell myself, "just do it." Maybe if I had taken my high heels off and put on Nikes and a jogging suit it would have been easier. But then people would have thought that this health-care executive was in need of a psychiatric consultation. (They might have been right anyway, no matter what my attire.) Over the next few days my office became a combination Hallmark store and florist shop. It made me feel really good that so many people cared that much about me.

I mentioned to a friend that only a few months before I had been eating lunch with a group from my department and we were discussing the recent death of the vice president of nursing service at the hospital. She had died of breast cancer, and it shocked every employee who knew her. She had been an oncology nurse for close to twenty years before being promoted to her VP position. People at the lunch table that day were stumped as to how she could have gotten breast cancer and then subsequently died from it. Even though everyone knew that the disease wasn't contagious, there was a mournful irony about her death because she had been a nurse in the field of medical oncology for such a long time. Then I spoke the words of doom to the group. "Breast cancer doesn't single out a particular type of person; it doesn't exclude any race. It doesn't focus in on people of a specific profession. It does not discriminate. It is a serious concern, or at least should be, for all women. There are twenty-eight women in our department. This means that if the statistics remain unaltered, three of us will develop breast cancer

sometime in our lifetimes." I must have looked like the Ghost of
Christmas Yet to Come from Dickens' *A Christmas Carol*. The
women looked at me with horror, as if I knew which three it would
be. Little did I know that the countdown to identifying the first of
the three would be known to us so soon.

The week that I pronounced those statistics, quite a few of the
staff who were over age forty called their doctors to get booked on
the mammogram schedule. You can be well-assured that anyone
who didn't get a mammogram then definitely signed up for one
when they heard I had been drafted as the first member of our
department to be enrolled in the "club."

I called the radiologist, Dr. Gayler, and told him the outcome of
my breast biopsy. I suggested that if the radiology department
wanted to have a two-for-one sale on boob pictures, this was the
week to do it. He, too, was surprised by my news. Despite the
appearance of the microcalcifications, what was hoped and
believed to be benign was not.

It was hard for me to decide whether to tell others at the hospital that I had breast cancer. At first I didn't want people to know
other than my own staff. Then I gave more thought to it and talked
with Al, and we decided that the more emotional support I had the
better off I would be. Plus, I needed to explain to people why I
would be moving my schedule around as well as why other staff
from my department would be attending meetings for me.

I wasn't prepared for some of the reactions. At times I wasn't
sure who was supporting and consoling whom. There were those,
mostly other nurses, who hugged me, showed their support, and
offered to do whatever would be helpful to me, whether at the hospital or at home. There were other folks who just disintegrated into
tears and needed consoling themselves. It definitely made me
aware of the vast number of people who associated this diagnosis
with death. And the recent death of our VP of nursing had probably further fostered those beliefs.

Then there were the people who had heard through the
grapevine that I was "sick." These poor unknowing souls were

caught completely off guard. One of them said to me, "I heard you were sick and were going to be in the hospital but that must have been a false rumor because you look great! Healthy as a horse!" When I responded by saying that the rumor wasn't all misinformation and that I was scheduled for surgery—and the kind of surgery it was—this person again said, "It's got to be a mistake. The doctor has made a mistake, Lillie, because you look fine."

Well, yes, it was true. I did look fine. Of course, most women who are diagnosed with breast cancer usually look fine. Even if I had been diagnosed in a much later stage of the disease, I imagine that I still would have looked peachy keen.

As I mentioned before, throughout my entire life I've looked healthy. Even when I've been very ill and at death's door I always seemed to look good immediately before and shortly thereafter. It did make me wonder what people (particularly those who don't have a medical background) thought someone with breast cancer should look like. Perhaps her bra would display a neon sign that would glow through her blouse to announce, "I'm sick and am going to be amputated soon." Maybe her affected breast would blow up twice the size of its mate and offer a clue that something was wrong.

Of course, showing no outward signs of disease is precisely why it's so important to go to the doctor each year for an examination. This is why it is necessary to do breast self-exams. This is why mammography is so valuable. It's because this disease is so subtle during its initial phases of establishing residency in a woman's breast. Cancer usually moves in quietly and without any fanfare. No trumpets blaring. No fever, no edema, no pain. It operates off squatter's rights and takes over whatever territory it pleases, and, if left unattended, takes over all of you.

I wanted my coworkers and others at the hospital to know the facts. I hoped that by sharing with them this very personal crisis I could gain the emotional support I needed to weather this fierce storm. I also hoped I could bring reality to the forefront and let people know that breast cancer could happen to anyone. I was an example of who "anyone" might be. I hoped that by being an example of this reality perhaps it would inspire others to not neglect the need to follow through with good preventive medical care—for themselves and for their sweethearts and other loved ones.

One gentleman who came by to see me when he heard the news was someone I had at least monthly contact with in meetings and weekly contact with by phone, as we handled a fair amount of business together. His concern for me was genuine and still is, although he had a major problem expressing it in the manner that I'm sure he had intended. As my husband would say, he had his tongue on top of his eye teeth and couldn't see what he was saying. The conversation went like this: "Lillie, I'm so sorry to hear about your bad news. How are you?" (He then glanced down at my chest.) "They look okay. I mean, you look okay. I've always thought they looked good. I mean, I've always thought that you looked good—healthy, I mean. Are you going to be okay? Are they going to go away? I mean, are you going to come back after your mastectomy?"

This poor man. His eyes were so fixed on my breasts that he couldn't get his eyes to come up to mine. The harder he tried the worse it got. I went into hysterics! I gave him a big hug and told him I was going to be okay. One of my breasts would go away and be replaced with an externally worn prosthetic one. The other one would still be around as far as I knew. He apologized for not being able to say correctly what he wanted to say. I told him that I really preferred the version that came out of his mouth. It lifted my spirits!

There was one person Al and I felt it was best not to tell over the phone or through someone else's voice. That was my grandmother. She was in her eighties, and we didn't feel it would be wise to telephone her as we had other family members. I knew the news would be a shock to her and we didn't want her to be unnecessarily worried. My grandfather had died just a few years before from prostate cancer. My great-grandfather had also died of the same. Both died in the house where she currently lived, and she had been their care taker until the end. Her association with cancer, for the most part, had been that cancer equals death. It would be important to dispel this image now.

So Al decided to go and pay her a visit while I was at work one day. He sat with her and told her what the situation was and emphasized that I would be fine. That I was going to be a survivor in the end. She took in every word. She believed what he said. Whether she believed it because of the way he said it or because she knew deep in her bones that it would be so, she believed—and that was all that mattered.

It was interesting to learn later that my mother had spoken to her on the phone before Al arrived at her house that day. My mother had told her the verdict, and grandmother, though upset to hear this news, remained convinced that I was going to do all right. I think that she had to convince my mother of this, curiously enough. Mom, at this point, was not dealing well with the situation herself. Fear of possibly losing me had overwhelmed her. The anxiety of having me undergo this kind of surgery gave her a migraine headache that would not go away.

Shirley and Jim, who are very dear friends of ours and have been for more than fifteen years, stopped by to see us the evening after Al called them on the phone. The four of us have helped each other through various and sundry crises. Each of us has had a turn. I was now up at bat again and they wanted us to know they were there for me and for Al. Shirley is a nurse and knew that I was well aware of what the surgery entailed and what other treatment might be lurking around the bend, depending on the outcome of my next pathology report from surgery.

Shirley is a good person to cry with. If ever you need a good cry, Shirley is a good friend to call. Having friends like this were very important to me. All so often in the past I would have closed people out of my life when the chips were down. This time, with my husband's encouragement, I wasn't going to do this. I was in a war with cancer and I needed as many people on my side as possible.

A key individual that I turned to, silently, in my own way, was God. I'm not the kind of person to run off to church and drop on my knees and say, "Take this away from me. Please. Give me something else. Something I can deal with, because I can't deal with this." I do pray, however, and do the majority of it at night, particularly when I'm restless and can't sleep. The house is quiet. My bedroom is dark. My thoughts are directed to my family, myself, the people I love. Just as there is an old cliché, "Be careful what you wish for," so I believe is the case with prayer. Be careful what you pray for.

Though I wondered why this had happened to me I didn't include it in any questions that I asked of God. I did ask him to let me live, to be a survivor of this medical experience, because I felt that I had more responsibilities and duties to be fulfilled here on earth. I also hoped that I was worthy of having the opportunity to have more pleasures from this world, too. Though that would certainly be his decision, I put in the request just the same.

One thing I knew for certain. This experience with breast cancer would change me for the rest of my life. Not just in the physical sense, but in the spiritual and emotional sense, too. Becoming a club member does that, I guess. No longer would I say "ho hum" when someone said to me that it was important to stop and smell the roses; that today is the first day of the rest of your life. I believe these sayings were written by club members who came before me. And I believe that their words came to have a very personal and profound meaning for me, one that warranted a moment of reflection and thought. These women were right. But their goal was not to be dead right.

On Saturday of the week I learned of my cancer, I was visited by another dear friend, Lynda, and her husband, Charles. They have known us a very long time. They've actually known my husband for more than twenty-five years and me for about fifteen of those. Lynda would often call me about various problems she was experiencing. Some related to the kids, some to work, some to other family crises. I'd lend an ear and try to help get her through with whatever support I could. I was always hesitant about reciprocating, though. For some reason I never wanted to bother anybody.

My troubles were mine and not to worry others with. However, Al had spoken to Lynda and Charles, and Lynda took time from her hectic schedule of housecleaning chores, baby-sitting grandchildren, and fixing meals to spend the day with me. She was a very powerful dose of spiritual medicine that day—probably more so than she will ever really know.

It is hard for me to describe Lynda to others. Anyone who has met her knows that she is unique. In some respects she is like a naive young girl, still learning about the world. In other ways, she is very wise. One thing you can count on—Lynda tells it like it is, and asks it like it is, too! That day she was on a special mission. Her mission was to get my spirits up and keep them there. She wanted me to erase from my mind all negative thoughts and think positively. Nothing else would be acceptable to her that day. When she arrived I was definitely down in a pit of gloom, and four hours later I, too, was convinced that I'd be okay. Better than okay. I'd turn this awful experience into something positive! How? Well, again, you are disadvantaged in that you don't know Lynda.

Lynda took me to Harryman House, a restaurant a few blocks away. We had a girls' lunch—something that rarely happened for either one of us. She proceeded to tell me what was on her mind and what she had discussed with Charles the night Al had called them with the news of my biopsy results.

"When Al called and said that it was cancer I just couldn't believe my ears. Then he said that you'd have to have a mastectomy. Oh no! But then I started thinking about it. Now let's see. What would I look like if one of my breasts were gone? So I went into the bedroom and took off my clothes and stood in front of the mirror and smashed down my left breast and I looked at myself. Then I bent over at the waist so my breasts were dangling in the air like pendulums from a clock, and tried to figure out how much my breast weighed. That's when Charles came in. He couldn't figure out what I was doing and thought I had lost my mind or something. Then I explained that I was making believe I was you and was trying to figure out what it would be like to have a breast gone. Well, I think that my breast weighs about three pounds. Of course I wasn't able to actually weigh it because I couldn't figure how to do that on the scale. But you know, Lillie, I think that you'll breathe better when it's gone! That breast is right over your heart and lungs, and I really do think that you'll breathe better, don't you?"

Well, as Lynda spoke and waved her hands to describe what she had done to demonstrate this science project of the hidden values of mastectomy surgery, I started laughing. I laughed and I laughed until tears ran down my face. What wonderful tears they were, too. Happy tears. Stress-reducing tears. And Lynda just looked at me trying to figure out why I found this description so funny, which is why Lynda is Lynda. She figured that everyone would have probably done the same thing that she did to simulate the experience of a mastectomy!

I'm sure there are other Lyndas out there. At least I hope so. We need more Lyndas so that those of us who are going through the real experience can appreciate the humor that someone who loves us dearly can bring to the forefront.

Lynda and I also had some time for more serious conversation. She was concerned about Laura's reaction to all of this. I told her that initially Laura seemed okay, but a few days later she wasn't. Several nights after I had my little talk with her I heard her crying in her room. When I went in to see what the matter was, she said that because I'd had complications when she was born that maybe whatever they were had caused these cancer cells to grow. She felt totally responsible and said that maybe if she had never been born I would be healthy now. It devastated me to hear these words. But I was thankful that at least she opened up to me and told me what was on her mind. I convinced her that her birth had nothing to do with this problem and that she was the best thing that ever happened to me.

Lynda wanted to reassure me that despite my concerns about my appearance, she knew Al was going to do fine. "It's only flesh. It's not you. Not the woman he married. He didn't marry you for your boobs. He loves you. And by the way, I want you to promise me that you'll show me your incision after your surgery. I want to see that battle scar. And I want to see your prosthesis, too. Everything!"

I took her picture outside on the deck before she went home that day. We talked for four hours straight. She'd ask me about what worried me and I'd tell her, and then she'd have some amazing one-liner that would put it into perspective. Her real message was to not let this thing get me. If I did, I'd be a goner. Stay on top of it. Stay optimistic. Seek the humor in the situation whenever possible, and remember that I am loved. She agreed that she, too, didn't think God was done with my stay on this earth. And she put me on her prayer list, and other people's prayer lists, too. That was very comforting.

I had the film developed the next day at a one-hour film processing store so that I could look at Lynda's face right away. Her picture stayed strategically placed on the coffee table for me to see every evening when I got home from work.

Another family we had always been close to was the Cross family, Pat and John. Though they lived several hours away from us, we saw them regularly and visited together as families. Al's daughter (from his previous marriage), Roxanne, viewed them as a second set of parents. There was even a time that Roxanne had lived with them, occupying an apartment they had fashioned for her in their basement when she was ready to start living more independently. Because Roxanne had married into a local family where the Crosses lived, we got to see them more often.

Pat and John had always been healthy people in general. Of course, so had we. The same time that I was served the verdict of breast cancer, John was given the verdict of brain cancer. He and I bonded together in a very special and unique way because we were going through troubled waters simultaneously. If you are going to be in a rowboat with no paddles and there is a hole in the boat, we decided that we'd gladly help each other bail. For Roxanne, it was very traumatic having two people she was very close to diagnosed with cancer. It was also very hard for Pat. What was happening made us all very much aware that cancer can affect anyone, even us.

One evening when Pat and John were visiting us we watched home videos that Pat had taken at our house the previous summer. As I looked at the video I realized that these people on film laughing and telling jokes and swimming in the pool really had nothing to be laughing about. They just didn't know it yet. I was looking at myself and John. Seemingly healthy on film, but both harboring cancer cells that would not make themselves known to us for several months to come.

So the resources I needed, the emotional ones, at least, were quickly being rounded up. My mother was rounding up even more of them behind the scenes. Work schedules were being reviewed and assignments to be divvied up were being prepared.

Chapter 7

My next plan of attack was to educate myself about breast cancer. Even though I was a nurse, I didn't feel like an expert when it came to the various kinds of breast cancer, the treatment options, and the research protocols currently in use. I wanted to be an expert, though, and fast. Over the weekend I went to the mall and ravaged the bookstores. I purchased *Dr. Susan Love's Breast Book.* I also got a few other books on cancer treatment modalities. On Friday, before coming home from work, I had been able to connect with Jean Wainstock, the breast cancer clinical nurse specialist that Dr. Yeo had told me about. She was very helpful and dropped off a lot of reading material about breast cancer published by the American Cancer Society.

I got home from the bookstores and promptly started reading. I couldn't put the material down. I felt better about what was going on in my life as long as I could read about it and remove some of the mystery and confusion about my future. Definitely the best money I ever spent was on Dr. Love's book. It also contained drawings, which I was able to share with my husband, that showed what the surgery—or at least the end result—would look like. All the information was important, and the author clearly understood how I was feeling. It was as if this book was for me and about me. It gave me peace of mind. It also served as a constant reminder that many women who were already club members had gone through this experience before me. In many cases their thoughts and feelings were echoes of my own.

I felt that information was power. I could perhaps gain some control over this experience if I was well-versed about the subject. I think I could have read all night the first night that I had this material in my hands. I didn't even stop to eat. Twice my husband asked me to give my eyes a break and come to the table, but I couldn't.

He compromised and fixed a plate for me and brought it into the living room. He, too, could see my energy level rising as I read more. He told me to mark any sections that I wanted him to read and that made me feel really good.

He was an instrumental player in this game of life and wanted to do whatever it took to have us both be winners. Many times he said to me that even though he was not the one with the diagnosis, he felt the pain, the anxiety, the fear. That's when I knew that we had a good marriage. If ever I had doubted it, this confirmed it for me. I could see in his face that this truly was our pain, our problem. I knew that with his strength, I could get myself on top of this dreadful thing and be a winner, a survivor.

Something else I did was to start scanning the Yellow Pages for mastectomy supplies. I wanted to learn everything. I became intrigued with the names of some of the shops that carried mastectomy bras, prostheses, swimwear, and other garments. They had names such as We Fit, Perfectly You, and Jodee's Inner Fashions. Very subtle names. It made me realize that to be an active member of this club you had to know the code words to figure out where to shop. I phoned one of the stores listed. The recording on their answering machine said they specialized in breast prostheses for use as external reconstruction to be worn during intimate moments. I thought that what they sold were perhaps stick-on boobs that had a battery-operated tassel hanging from a fake nipple. You could flick a switch and get the tassel to go clockwise, or if your husband preferred, counterclockwise. I ended up visiting their shop at a later time and was disappointed to find that what their advertisement referred to was the creation of a breast prosthesis made from a mold taken from your other breast. It was very expensive, too. Close to $1,600. I would have preferred not having had my fantasy shattered and wished I had never paid them a visit. Oh well. Perhaps if Blaze Star has a friend who ever gets breast cancer, she will create such a line of prosthetic gadgets and call her shop Blaze's Boobery Boutique. I might even consider stopping in there for a novelty item for a special occasion.

Al surprised me Sunday evening by buying crabs. It was a hard decision to put my reading material down, but the smell of steamed crabs did the trick. He was right. I needed a break. I had read more than 400 pages of material in two days without skimming over anything. And I had learned the material well enough to recite just about any section back to him verbatim. He won me over, however, with the crabs. I love steamed crabs. He told me that he had enough money on him to buy me one-and-a-half-dozen roses or two dozen steamed crabs. He chose wisely—he knew me well. Crabs were far more romantic to me that day than flowers ever would have been.

On Monday it was back to the old grindstone. Work was very good for me. It kept my mind off my troubles, at least most of the time, and it made me feel productive.

That morning in the shower I realized that I seemed to be avoiding touching my left breast. I'd rub the bar of Coast soap all over me but there. At first I hadn't been touching it because of the biopsy incision that was still tender, but that was no longer the case. There was what seemed to be purposeful avoidance, and even though I was aware of it, I wasn't able to do anything about it. I felt as if this part of my body wasn't deserving of good hygiene. It was infected with something bad and that perhaps touching it would encourage it to spread. Even though I knew this was a silly thought, I still avoided it. I also avoided looking in mirrors when I got out of the shower. Avoidance was my defense mechanism, and I maintained it, generally speaking, until my surgery date. I didn't even bother to look at how well, or not well, my incision was healing. Why bother? It was healing only long enough to be cut off anyway and discarded. I wondered if after the mastectomy, some medical student would be given my breast to examine and study the stages of tissue healing after surgery. That was about all that this biopsy/lumpectomy incision was good for now.

I chuckled to myself on occasion about how upset I had been when I first came home from my outpatient surgery and saw the three-and-a-half-inch incision. To think that I was worried and distressed about how my breast looked post-op. The joke was surely on me now. I realized that I should have been thrilled to have only a three-and-a-half-inch incision dimpling my breast. I remembered when I said my prayers in those weeks before surgery that I had learned a valuable lesson. The lesson was to be grateful for what I had and not wish for something more than what had been given to me. It was a hard pill to swallow, but a lesson that would last me a lifetime. At least I hoped it would.

The nights were the hardest for me. Even after my prayers I would still find myself sobbing. Al would hold me very tightly. He didn't say much. That was best. No words were needed. I just couldn't believe that this was happening to me. It continued to feel like a bad dream. I would tell myself that if ever I woke up and confirmed that this was all a dream, I'd never eat before bedtime again. (Frequently, I'd have a bowl of cereal before bedtime, and when I did I almost always had nightmares or bizarre dreams of some kind. If I ever woke up from this experience, Cheerios were going to be banned from the house.)

I decided that it would be smart to see my psychotherapist more often between this time and my surgery date, so we had weekly sessions. Marla was helpful in letting me express things that I was afraid to say out loud even when I was by myself. She served as a good person to bounce information off and make sure that I really wasn't losing my mind, just my breast.

One of my two bosses, Chip, came by for an unexpected visit during the week. He had been told of my situation by Tim and wanted to show his support. It was hard for him to express his emotions, but that was okay. I had known Chip for more than a decade, and what emotions he showed me that day were more than I would ever have expected. He reassured me that I was in good hands with the medical and surgical team there at the hospital. These words weren't necessary. I had confidence in my doctors. Still, it was nice to have it reaffirmed.

I concentrated much of my time on making short-term and long-term plans for my office. Planning all of the "what-ifs." You know, what if I need to be out longer than a month? How should I divvy up the workload? What if there are complications and I need to be out longer or need chemotherapy? It was very important to me not to leave any loose ends. I didn't want to be a burden to anybody. I also didn't want to return to chaos. My staff, especially Scott, Marge, Bryanna, Joyce, and Sheila, and of course Diane, were super. "You just tell us what you want us to do and we'll do it," they said. It was easier to hear those words than it was to figure out how to reallocate the work. Projects that I was half-way through I wanted to have wait until I was able to finish them myself. Decisions that needed to be made at a director's level would either have to be punted to Tim or wait for my return. It was complicated. I decided that if at all possible I would have work brought home to me after my first week or so while I recuperated. So that's how we left it. Assignments were given, work flow rearranged, and a schedule prepared. It felt awkward, but very necessary just the same.

I knew that I had about two weeks or so left before going on vacation, followed upon my return by surgery. My transformation surgery. The surgery that would, hopefully, transform me from a breast cancer victim into a breast cancer survivor.

Most days at work, time really raced by, but at night it inched itself along. Nights fell into a steady pattern of eating dinner, reading any new material that I'd been able to get my hands on about breast cancer and its treatment, reviewing whatever documents I had brought home from work to complete, then going to bed for a restless night. I'd get to bed and within about twenty minutes start crying. Al would hold me or rub my back and I'd cry. The living nightmare continued for weeks.

Chapter 8

Here it was summertime and I wasn't having the time of my life, as I'd expected. We had been planning a Hawaiian party at our house for weeks, but now I was undecided if we should cancel it because of these new developments in our lives. I wanted people to have a good time. It was a party, not a funeral. But I didn't know if I could have a good time or not. Gee, I certainly didn't want to go on a crying jag right in front of everybody. The majority of the folks we had invited were people from the hospital, and crying would have been very embarrassing. Instead of handing out Hawaiian leis, I would be handing out Kleenex. Not good. So we gave it a lot of careful thought.

The conclusion we reached was that this party would be one of the best things we could do for ourselves. To be surrounded by friends who are also work associates, and to have a happy time! So the party plans stayed intact. Not everyone who had been invited was aware of my present health status, so I decided to send out some special notes to those who would not have heard the news yet. My mistake was in sending these documents to their work addresses, not realizing that some were out of town and wouldn't be back at work to review their mail until after the party. My intentions were to have no one surprised by the news in the event that someone brought it up. I did, however, request of the attendees that people avoid the subject for the day. This was to be a party! A time to relax, eat, drink, swim, tell funny stories, and enjoy each other's company. Hugs were welcome. It was not a pity party.

And it worked out great! Everyone had a good time, including me. We laughed and talked and ate until we were all ready to explode. I didn't know that several of our guests (Haya, Albert, and Earl) had not received my personal notes and were unaware of the circumstances at hand. I just thought that they were being polite and respectful of my request to not discuss the subject. But I could tell by some of their comments that they were still in the dark. Particularly when they were discussing work-related projects and things that we would be working on together in the middle of July, which at that time was still a few weeks away. I didn't listen to the details of the projects being discussed because I knew that I would be working on my own project. My project of being transformed from a cancer victim into a cancer survivor. Certainly to be the most important project of my life to date.

We decided to invite my parents to the party. We wanted to visit with them, give them an opportunity to meet some of my colleagues, and see me in a happy mood. We hoped that maybe the party would lift their spirits, too. Dad and Mom arrived early to visit with us before the gang arrived. This was the first time they had seen me since my diagnosis was made known to them, and they needed some time alone with me. My mother looked ten years older to me in a period that in actuality covered only two to three weeks. She was really having a hard time of it. I felt awful for her. I was the cause of her looking so sad, so worried, and there was nothing I could do to make it magically go away. Of course that was what she needed—for it to magically go away and have me all better again. I was careful that day not to succumb to the overwhelming feeling to just sit down with her and go on a major crying jag. But I stayed focused on the party, the food preparation, and the necessity to have a fun day.

My father camped out for a while in the living room, alone. When I finished fixing the food trays I went in to him. Mom was occupied with Laura, being caught up on who her latest boyfriend was. When I entered the living room, I found Dad with his eyes fixed on the open pages of *Dr. Susan Love's Breast Book*. He appeared ill. He was looking at the drawings of the mastectomy incision post-op. He looked up at me and started crying. This was a surprise to me. My dad wasn't the kind to show emotion. He always wanted to present himself as a tough guy. He really isn't, though. He just doesn't like to admit it. Looking at the book upset him. It put the problem into a very physical one, and one that was too close for comfort for him. He didn't know what to say and was distressed with himself that I had found him crying. I told him that I was going to be okay and that I wanted this to be a good day, a fun day for everyone. He responded as he often did in a family crisis. "I know. If you need anything, just buy it. Your mother is going to put money in a joint account for you. Spend it. Medical bills will come in fast now. I don't want you to want for anything and go without because you don't have the money to pay for things you need."

He was right. Dad frequently talked about money. It was a major part of his upbringing; it was a major focal point in my mother's life, too. Dad, I think, associated money with security, and he wanted me to be secure. He wanted to provide me with protection, even if the only protection he could give me right now was financial protection. He knew he couldn't rid me of this problem by giving money to someone to put a magic spell on me and make my breast disease-free overnight. However, he didn't want me to shortchange myself from receiving the best medical treatment that money could buy, nor did he want me to be distracted with monthly bills in the event that I had to be off from work for an extended period of time. He knew that I was the breadwinner in the family; that my husband had been laid off from work several years earlier on a medical disability because of a back problem.

What Dad didn't know was that I thought as he did, or perhaps, better phrased, as he and Mom had taught me. I had a lot of sick time built up, plus I had good health-care insurance coverage. I also had additional short-term and long-term disability insurance in the event of a medical problem like this. So I felt financially stable, at least for the time being. His gesture was genuine and it was his way of showing me that he wanted me well. It was also his way of saying that he loved me.

The party went off without a hitch—at least, almost without a hitch. Toward the end of the day when people were preparing to leave, I saw Haya talking with my mother. My mother looked very teary-eyed, and I sensed that she had decided to take a moment to talk with Haya about her concerns for me. Haya was a physician and someone my mother had spent time with before, so it was natural for my mother to talk with her in private. Shortly after their conversation, my folks left and headed back to their farm on the eastern shore. For the rest of the evening, Haya frequently glanced over at me and smiled, but looked perplexed.

When she was ready to leave, she asked if she could have a word with me. We took a brief stroll down the sidewalk. She told me that my mother seemed very upset and not herself, and when she had inquired what was troubling her, my mother had responded by saying she was worried about me. Worried that she would lose me. Frustrated that she couldn't control the situation. My mother hadn't explained what the situation was, however. That's when I figured out that Haya hadn't gotten my letter. She had been out of town and hadn't seen her mail yet. I paused a moment. First I thought that I'd simply tell her to wait and read her mail. Then I realized this would not have been a fair answer. I had almost gotten through the afternoon without a mention of my problem. And that felt good. For a while, I had been able to fantasize that it was only a dream. Here I stood before a friend who knew that something strange was going on but had no idea what. I finally got up the nerve to tell her. "I've been diagnosed with breast cancer." Where are the Kleenex when you need them? We both burst into tears. She, like so many others, offered her support. Being a doctor herself she instinctively began asking me medical questions about my treatment plan. She also said she knew that neither Albert nor Earl knew about my medical problem, and she offered to give them a status report of my situation. It was an emotionally labile day.

Why was this happening to me? I used to think when I was little that God had this big book the size of my father's cow barn. In this book were two pages for each person on earth. On one page he put down check marks when you did something really good; on the other side he'd record check marks when you were really bad. When you died he'd add up the check marks. If the number of good check marks outnumbered the number of bad check marks, then you would have a place with him beyond the pearly gates. If you didn't, you would go to a place that was really awful and full of demons. (I guess if I had been a child of the nineties I would have had God use a calculator or computer to keep score.)

As an adult, I had developed different views on the subject. Perhaps God kept a different kind of scoring system. Perhaps he had a big matrix chart on each person divided into various categories, which included good experiences and bad experiences. He assigned a grade to our performance with each experience. For example, if you had a good experience like having a baby, maybe he evaluated your performance as a mother. Were you loving, kind, caring, nurturing, and so on? (I realize that some people reading this would have categorized the same experience as a bad one.) If a bad experience is receiving a diagnosis of breast cancer, what are his criteria for measuring our performance? Does he evaluate how well we deal with body disfigurement? Is it perhaps a test of our marriage vows that say, "for better, for worse, in sickness and in health?" If so, I wanted to get a good score! I wanted to stay on top of this thing and not let it get me. I wanted him to see that I had faith and could deal with it, no matter what the long-term outcome would be. This was just a piece of flesh and not really me, not my mind, and certainly not my soul. My goal was to be a breast cancer survivor, and to become one I would do whatever was asked of me. I wanted to get an A+ in this matrix box.

Chapter 9

On Father's Day, June 21 that year, we called my dad to wish him a happy Father's Day. Unfortunately Dad was out, so we weren't able to talk to him. Mom was home by herself and having as she termed it "a bad day." She was very tearful and had apparently been crying before she even heard my voice on the phone. She kept saying that she "wanted a miracle" and that she had contacted many churches and asked that my name be placed on their prayer lists. She wanted to reach someone who knew Mother Seton. She was very upset—perhaps best described as angry. Distressed that she had no control over what was happening to her child. Feeling helpless. Wanting a miracle to occur that would rid me of this awful thing. No words that I spoke seemed to comfort her that day.

I felt awful for her and for myself. I tried to reassure her that I would be all right but she just couldn't accept that as an answer. She kept telling me that this wasn't supposed to be happening to me. I'd had enough things go wrong in my life and that this was wrong for it to be happening to me. She wanted it to be her. She told me that if this was her breast she'd feel okay about it. She could deal with that. She couldn't accept it because it was happening to me instead of her. I told her repeatedly that it was neither her choice nor her fault. No one had pulled my name out of a hat and said that I win the booby (cancer) prize. I also told her that I felt relieved that of the two of us it was me, because I was in a better state of physical and emotional health to deal with it.

Al also tried to comfort her but it seemed useless that day. This was a woman who would walk through fire for her family, but this time there was no fire to walk through to take the problem away and remove the hurt and emotional pain.

My mother has always been a very active member of the church, perhaps even recognized as, I'd say, a pillar of the church, yet she was somehow not receiving the peace of mind she so desperately needed at this moment. Her insistence to contact Mother Seton surprised me because we're not even Catholic! I started thinking that perhaps much of the problem was that she felt trapped. Trapped between two generations that had been stricken with cancer. Her father had died of prostate cancer, which was a very painful experience for her. She and I stood together at his bedside in her parents' home when he took his last breaths. He was alert until the end and did not want to die. I believe his life was extended by a few days because of my mother's presence. He wanted to be with her and fought off the closing of death's door for as long as he could.

Now she was looking at the generation coming after her—her own child—and feared she would once again be placed in a situation that was all too familiar. Her fear of its potential threat overwhelmed her and challenged her to gain control in any way that she could. Prayer was a very constructive way, and I was glad she sought that path.

After that day it was reassuring to know when I went to bed at night that many people across the state of Maryland, and even in nearby states, were asking God to take care of me (and perhaps grade me on a curve).

On weekends I spend a lot of time running errands and shopping. If there is a bargain to be had I can sniff one out. I even think that I might possess a special bargain shopping gene that God gave me when I was born. I figure that he gave it to me, personally, because no one else in my family has this trait. I'm the kind of person most Christmas shoppers hate because I usually finish my Christmas shopping as early as four weeks after New Year's Day. And I can do it for about a fraction of what others spend during the actual shopping season. Now, however, the shopping malls started to take on a different image for me.

I started doing what I so well-remembered my brother doing when he was a teenager and young adult and we went shopping together: I started looking at women's breasts. I felt compelled to.

I looked at each woman at the mall and tried to figure out if I could spot an experienced member of the club. I'd look to see if a woman's breasts bounced when she walked. If they did, I assumed that they were real and that the woman wasn't in the breast cancer survivors' club.

Then I would look at people thinking they might be future draftees. I'd count the women as they walked by...one, two, three, four, five, six, seven, eight! Oh no! She might be the next one! And she probably doesn't even know it! Oh, the poor dear! No matter how many women I saw or where I saw them, I wondered if I was secretly in the presence of the post-mastectomy patient. It was really nutty, but that's what I did.

Poor Al. When he was with me, I'd ask for his opinion, too. "What do you think of that set over there? The one on the right doesn't seem to bounce as much as the one on the left. Do you agree?" He'd just shrug his shoulders and walk on down the aisles with me. Clearly I should have had my brother with me because he was a real boob man. He'd know the answers for sure. But, alas, he was living in Japan.

Sometimes Laura would be out shopping with me. We'd be at a mall or in the grocery store together and I'd ask her to help me locate a woman who might be wearing a fake boob. She didn't want to play this game. That was clear. And she usually walked in the other direction. Perhaps she was afraid of what I would do if I was successful in my search. Maybe she thought I would ask to touch it or something. I never did find one. Despite my routine explorations, I came up empty-handed, so to speak, convinced that if I were seeing other breast cancer survivors who'd had a mastectomy, all of them must have had reconstruction.

Although arrangements had been made for me through the hospital for a Reach to Recovery volunteer to come see me after my surgery, I longed to talk to someone now, before the deed was done. So I called the Reach to Recovery office and asked to speak with a current breast cancer survivor who'd had a mastectomy under the age of forty and was married. It became clear to me that the organization was not used to receiving calls directly from patients and that it did not usually connect volunteers with anyone until the patient was in the post-op state.

I wanted to talk with someone about what I should expect upon waking up, and about other personal matters like intimacy with your mate, and I wanted to talk NOW—not two weeks from now. In two weeks I would be able to answer most of the questions now burning in my mind by doing a self-retrospective evaluation of my own recovery room experience. So the woman who answered the phone agreed to have a volunteer call me back. I also requested that the volunteer be a large-busted woman. I felt that talking to a woman who wore a size 32AA bra before her surgery was not in the same boat with me, the wearer of a 42D cup. That was an important patient mix variable in my book.

Two days later I did receive a call from a volunteer. She was fairly helpful but I didn't feel as connected to her emotionally as I had hoped to be. She was a 34A.

I also had a major concern about some other medical management issues that related to my short-term and long-term survival. These issues surrounded the kind of anesthesia I would be receiving. I'd had a bad track record with general anesthesia in the past. At the age of thirteen, I'd had an emergency appendectomy and had intraoperative complications from anesthesia. As a result my blood pressure bottomed out and my recovery time in the recovery room was extended by three hours. When I was in labor with Laura and a vaginal delivery attempt was unsuccessful, an emergency C-section was done. I demanded not to be put to sleep because of my reaction to general anesthesia so a rapid spinal anesthesia was given. Unfortunately, I had trouble with it as well and awoke in the ICU because of respiratory failure. This pattern repeated itself again after I had urgent surgery for abdominal adhesions and ovarian cyst removal.

Needless to say, the thought of general anesthesia was a major concern to me. I didn't want to be one of the cases about which the doctor comes out of the O.R. and says, "the operation was a success, but the patient died."

So I started figuring out what I could do to try and influence the odds in my favor. I decided to get advice from Tim, hoping that he could help me get connected with an appropriate physician in the anesthesia department who could look out for me during the surgery.

One thing in my favor was that this surgery was taking place in a controlled environment. What I mean is that I wasn't having this procedure done as an emergency operation, like a patient with a gunshot wound does. Each time I had experienced trouble it had been during and immediately following emergency surgery. Another thing in my favor was that I was in a position to make a special request for a particular anesthesiologist because of my role in the hospital. I'm sure that all of the anesthesiologists were excellent, but again I was seeking control.

Tim offered to talk with the chief of the anesthesiology department and explain my past medical history. I was unable to get any of my medical records from previous hospitalizations, so we had to go with historical information that I provided. It would have been best to have the records so they could see what drugs I had been given, but that was not possible.

I asked Tim to ask the following question of the Chief of the Sandmen Gang. "If I were the Chief's wife (assuming he loves his wife), who would he recommend put her to sleep knowing this specific medical history with anesthetic agents." He did ask. The answer was Dr. Charles Beattie.

Dr. Beattie called me that same day and introduced himself. He reviewed with me my medical history, surgical/anesthetic events, and what kind of allergies I have. Since the last time I'd had surgery ten years earlier, many new and improved drugs had come on the market and were being used along with some of the more standard anesthesia agents. Dr. Beattie arranged for me to be examined, and for chest X-rays and some other tests to be done. He also wanted to get a special view of my neck, because it is part of my medical history that I have a narrow airway (I have a multi-nodular goiter). He was wonderful. I could tell by his voice and the depth of his medical evaluation that I was in excellent hands. Anesthesia was still a worry, but not as severe a worry as it had been.

As the day neared, Laura started spending more time with me. Instead of spending time in her room listening to her cassette tapes blaring, she spent it with me. We'd watch a funny movie or play Wheel of Fortune on the computer. She has always been an affectionate child, but it was clear that her concerns for my survival and well-being rested heavily on her mind. "I love you Mommy." I heard this phrase at least six times a day. "Even though you say you will be different after your surgery, I don't think you will really change. You'll be the same to me and that's all that matters to me." What comforting words to hear from someone so young.

Al also tried to provide me with constant reassurance that he would still love me. My breast's absence wouldn't make a bit of difference to him. He kept telling me this, especially at night when we were in bed. He kept saying it, but I was afraid to believe it.

"You don't understand yet what my incision is going to look like. You can't tell me that it won't make a difference until you see it. Then we'll both see for real how you feel." I told him it might be months before I'd let him even see my incision.

He said that would be my decision but I was worrying about nothing. He said he respected my wishes. He added, "Well, that will be up to you. After all, you've never seen me without my teeth in. I'm funny about that, you know."

We chuckled about that. We'd been married almost fifteen years and in all that time I had never seen him without his upper plate in. He slept with his upper plate in, too. I told him that maybe I'd make a deal with him. He could show me his toothless smile and I'd show him my one-breasted chest. He thought that seemed like a fair deal. I told him he needn't worry about having to practice his smile for awhile because I didn't think I'd be ready for several weeks after my surgery; possibly even several months. He told me he'd wait for the signal from me.

Chapter 10

On the weekend of June 29, my brother, his wife, and their two children came to visit us. They had come home from Japan for a vacation. Robert, Mary, and kids (Julie age eleven, and David age seven) had been in Japan for nearly three years. My brother was a colonel in the Air Force—one of those crazed people who like to travel through the air as if their hair were on fire. That's why he's such a good F16 pilot.

They hadn't been home for a year. This vacation visit with us was a strained one because of the circumstances of my health. When I had gotten the diagnosis originally, I couldn't even talk with them on the phone. Just to hear Robert ask me, "How're you doing, Sis?" completely disintegrated me to tears. I had done a lot of practicing, talking about my surgical treatment plans, before they actually came home. By the time they arrived, I was able to discuss it as if it were happening to someone else. A coping mechanism, I guess.

Robert didn't ask me directly about anything related to my health. Mary did most of the questioning. During this vacation she was surrounded by breast cancer. Mary's mother also had breast cancer and had deferred surgical intervention. Her folks live in Colorado, and she and my brother would be traveling to see Mary's folks after spending time with us and with my parents on the farm.

We spent our time together swimming in the pool, eating crabs, and watching our children play together. The kids really missed one another. This was a special time to witness the value of a close family unit. Lots of pictures were taken. Robert didn't need to say too much to me. It wasn't necessary. He's never wanted to dwell on sad situations. He'd rather not discuss it, focusing mostly on neutral topics. His concern was genuine, but a lot of conversation on the subject wasn't really needed between us. Often in the past when he had been home to visit, we'd talk very little.

Robert did tell me that he had been seen by the flight surgeon for a growth in his throat—the same kind that Mom and I had each been diagnosed with and treated for. The link for the three of us was the same. These growths are believed to be caused by exposure to strong chemicals—the pesticides and insecticides that Dad had used for years on the crops. Apparently the way these used to be mixed and sprayed on the ground was the same mixture and method used during the Vietnam War to spread Agent Orange. The ingredients were the same chemical compound. It made us all thankful that our children hadn't been born with birth defects. However, it did raise the question as to whether this contributed to my present condition. We realized there had already been some effects since all three of us had abnormal tissue that had grown in our throats.

My father became very sentimental during the visit with Rob and his family at our house. He had mailed me a personal letter about ten days before Rob arrived home. This was a rare thing for Dad to do. It was filled with words of love and emotion. I was surprised and impressed that he mentioned that letter to Rob and Mary while we were eating crabs. He was definitely wanting to make sure that the things that had been left unsaid in the past were said now, and said often. From that day on, including up to now, whenever I see Dad, he always makes sure to tell me he loves me.

These were words not frequently used by him before that time. It was the beginning of a new relationship between us and it felt good. Our relationship was closer because my body was betraying me and flirting with death. God truly did bring some positive moments into a very bad experience. Moments that would last for the rest of my life. Our family's goal was for that time frame to be a very long one.

Two days after Robert and Mary left our home, Al and I were on a plane for our vacation. Laura went with Robert and his family over to the farm to continue her visit with her cousins, whom she missed so very much. Though our vacation had been planned for months in advance, my enthusiasm about the trip was gone. We were going to one of my very favorite places—Maine. I had planned to stuff myself with lobster until I couldn't stand looking at those big red crustaceans anymore. But now I just didn't feel like it. I knew that when we came back home it would be time for my mastectomy. I wanted to trade in our round-trip tickets for a one-way and just stay there. Forget about all of this mess. Just sit by the ocean and listen to the waves crashing and the lighthouse horn sounding in the distance. I again felt like Dorothy in *The Wizard of Oz*. The hourglass had been turned over and my time was running out. I wondered if I would feel better if I bought a pair of red-sequined shoes. Probably not. I didn't know how to make them work anyway. And they'd be expensive and probably not on sale.

I decided to do all my packing at once and get it out of the way. One suitcase for Maine, one small bag for the hospital. I also switched my watch that day from my left wrist to my right. An odd thing to do, you might think, but I knew that after surgery it would need to be on the right side in the future, probably permanently. That's because with a left-sided mastectomy, some of the lymph nodes are removed from the left armpit areas (axilla). This can result in arm edema. Some people keep the edema for a long time. After any kind of strenuous activity some people have experienced swelling of their arms. It is unwise to wear anything that constricts on the arm affected by the surgery. So I decided I might as well start getting used to wearing my watch on the other wrist. That way there would be one less adjustment in the future.

Unfortunately, this adjustment served as a constant reminder that my days of being a two-breasted woman were numbered. From habit I was constantly looking at my left wrist to check the time. When I realized I had switched it, a shroud of gloom would come into my mind and I'd think about why I was looking at the wrong wrist. I'm a constant clock watcher and have been all my life, so this feeling of gloom was ever-present. But I left the watch on its new wrist just the same.

We left for Maine as planned. On the plane I worried that I might have gotten mixed up and packed our camera in the wrong suitcase. That would have been interesting—taking a camera into the operating room. Ugh...I had placed it in the right bag after all, so it was a minor worry. I also packed my diary (which my psychotherapist friend, Marla, had recommended I keep and take with me to record my thoughts and feelings.)

For reading material, I brought along a book written by a breast cancer survivor. She'd had a mastectomy when she was young, too. I hoped it would be uplifting and give me a feeling of hope and support, particularly since I was now reading the last half of the book, which concentrated on her life six months to eight years after her mastectomy. But the book didn't lift me up at all. It made me feel worse.

Here was a single woman who published the fact that even after reconstructive surgery, she didn't have sex for five and a half years! She wrote that men rejected her. Good heavens. What a sad thing to share with the world. I wanted to read about a woman in her thirties who had done well after her surgery—physically, emotionally, and spiritually. This was not a woman who would serve as a role model for me. I felt sorry for her. She must have kept running into and subsequently dating some real jerks. Then I realized that I had been out of the dating game for fifteen years. I was married. It made me very thankful to be married. Dating is difficult enough. It must be an awful challenge to date someone and have to make the awkward decision about when to tell him that you've had a mastectomy. "Hi. My name is Lillie. I'm a Libra. I've got one boob. What's your name?"

Yes. I was among the fortunate. At least I hoped that I was. If Al had trouble adjusting to my physical state of being after my surgery, what would I do? What would he do? He'd been reassuring me that he would be fine with it. But the real test had not come yet. We talked a lot about that specific issue. How did Al know he would be fine about it? He hadn't seen what I would look like, so how could he possibly know that a giant scar across my chest wouldn't be a turn-off for him? He just continually repeated that he "knew."

I felt like taking him to a horror flick and watching his facial reactions while various grotesque monsters suddenly appeared on the screen. Then I realized that I wasn't being fair to my surgeon. For all I knew, his needle work would look so good that even I wouldn't feel offended by what I saw. The fact of the matter was, however, that at this moment in time I just didn't know. I could only speculate.

When Al and I had private time and were in intimate situations I usually cried, both during and after. I couldn't get out of my mind that this wonderful, loving, and tender relationship we had was about to be abolished by a scalpel. It really scared me. Once I got the definitive diagnosis of breast cancer, he stopped touching me above the waist when we were in bed. I was relieved, but sometimes I misinterpreted it as his practicing to never touch my breasts again. Gee, I'll still have one left. Will it be off limits because its partner is about to be evicted from the premises for demonstrating unacceptable behavior? I felt it best to not discuss it. I'd just let time take its course and determine our future private relationship.

One evening when we were sitting on the balcony of our room in Bar Harbor, Al and I were talking about how long I anticipated my recovery to take. I had hoped about four weeks or so.

I talked about a patient I had taken care of once who'd been admitted for a GI workup. Several years before that she'd had a mastectomy. A very nice woman, she was in her fifties at the time I met her. She was married to a wonderful man, whom I had met as well. It was obvious that they had a really special relationship.

I had gotten up the nerve to ask her some questions about her breast cancer experience. I asked her how long it took her to adjust to her breast being gone. Her reply was a surprising one to me. She said on some days, she didn't feel like it was gone. That's because she had a phantom limb sensation. Just like amputees who lose a leg or an arm, she had the sensation that her breast was still there. She even told me that she enjoyed having her husband touch her incision in certain spots because it simulated the pleasant feeling that she used to have when her breast was there.

She absolutely shocked me when she said she thought that the nerve that went to her nipple was stitched somewhere in the sutures that were sewn in her armpit, because she loved her husband to kiss her there! I must have looked like a very shocked and naive young woman to her that day. She said, "You might be a nurse in your early twenties, but I can tell that you haven't had much experience in the world yet." She was right about that. I had been too embarrassed to talk any more about it.

Now, on that night in Bar Harbor seventeen years later, I would have given a lot of money to find that lady so I could talk with her again. Al seemed intrigued and very attentive while I told him this story. He didn't laugh, though I did. He told me that this could be my story in the near future, and I might be telling someone about our experiences yet to come. He said, "I'll nibble on your elbow, armpit, neck, anywhere!"

About a half-hour later as we were going back to our room for the night, he said, "Just one question. There's no chance that your nipple nerve could end up in your rear end, is there? I love you, but I might have to draw the line there." We had a big laugh over that. I assured him that it would stay somewhere in the region of the incision. I also told him that not every woman had phantom limb sensation after a mastectomy.

On our last night of vacation, I felt well-rested and much more at ease with my situation, though I must admit my mood was very changeable. The weather had not been very good during part of our trip, but we'd enjoyed each other's company. I appreciated the sun when it was shining and even admired the sudden changes in the weather when a thunderstorm blew in. I had rarely ever taken the time to look at the sky except when the weather was nice. I was learning to value all of the weather now because it meant that I was alive. I was here. I wasn't pushing up daisies from six feet under. I was finally learning to stop and smell the roses.

Our last night was spent in Portland. Before we were ready to go to bed, we decided to catch the last half of a show on TV. I don't know if it was *Prime Time Live* or *20/20*, but it was great. Just what we both needed. The show was about a baseball player who had bone cancer, which eventually resulted in his losing his entire arm and shoulder. It was his left arm, his pitching arm.

He and his wife were each interviewed. Each talked about how this tragic experience changed their lives, but in the long run it had changed for the better. Sure, he wished it had never happened to him. Sure, it resulted in his not being able to play major league baseball anymore. But he talked about the positive things that had occurred because of it.

It strengthened their marriage, it gave them both an appreciation for life, and it brought them closer to God. Now his time was spent on lecture circuits talking about his experience. He had met a lot of children who hadn't been as fortunate as he. These were kids who also had cancer but would eventually, in some instances, be swiftly swept from this earth and taken from the people who loved them—their parents, their sisters and brothers, their grandparents, their little friends. It gave him a new perspective about life and about the value of it.

He said he believed that God had given him this tragedy so he could instill hope into other cancer victims. I didn't know whether this was so—whether God gave this to him, I mean. I did know about the other part though, because he instilled hope in me that night. He didn't have breast cancer, but he had lost a part of his body that he valued very much. It was directly connected to his livelihood, too. He went on with his life and was clearly a better person for it. Al turned to me and said, "That will be us very soon."

Chapter 11

I went into work for just a day or so after vacation and before my surgery date. I wanted to clear up any burning items that needed to be handled so I would truly feel that I was starting with as clean a slate as possible when my surgical sick leave began. I also had an appointment in the Same Day Surgery Center to have a pre-operative evaluation and get my chest X-ray, blood work, and such completed. At that time the big day was only two days away.

I also saw Dr. Yeo (Charlie), and he reviewed the specifics of the surgery with me and my post-operative recovery regimen. He had me sign a surgical consent form, which plainly told what the surgery was, why it was being done, and what the risks were. I signed it, trying to keep my cool and not cry as my pen marked the paper with my signature.

I had planned to ask some questions about exactly what my incision would look like, but I became too nervous. It was probably just as well. No sense in dwelling on this subject longer than absolutely necessary.

Charlie had previously discussed with me the option of having reconstructive surgery done at the same time. Although I was not a candidate for implants, I was a candidate for a tram flap procedure. Because I had opted against having that done, he explained that not choosing this additional procedure didn't mean I had burned my bridges; I could opt to have this done in the future. He mentioned that some plastic surgeons actually prefer that patients wait six months before the second procedure. In that way the healing process is optimal. I had very mixed feelings about this procedure and a great concern about being under anesthesia for eight to ten hours. I also didn't know if I wanted my abdominal flesh and vessels relocated onto my chest. It might look like a breast mound, but my brain would know it wasn't. Anyway, I was glad that this option wasn't a do-it-now-or-you-lose-your-chance kind of procedure.

Dr. Yeo explained that I would be going home about twenty-four hours after the operation and would be taking home two hemovacs, or wound-draining devices. Because I was a nurse, I was already familiar with these devices, so no detailed explanation was needed.

Shortly before I'd gone on vacation, I'd sent Dr. Yeo a personal note thanking him for the time he had spent with me on the phone, letting him know that I knew I was in good hands. I'd also drawn a silly cartoon on the card for him, letting him know that I wasn't going to let this experience rob me of my sense of humor. He was very amused by my drawing and appreciative of my card. That made me feel really good. (I had realized after I sent the card to him that he might think I was some kind of nut. But I was willing to run that risk to let him know more about me and my style of handling medical crises.)

I have opted to draw for you the same cartoon, or should I say riddle, that I had drawn for him.

Question: What is this a picture of?

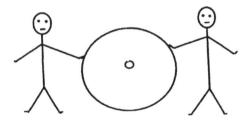

Answer: It's two men walking "abreast."

Now is that funny, or what? I sure thought so, and fortunately, Charlie did too.

I realized that this physician was going to be—and had already become—a very important person in my life. He was the individual able to transform me from a cancer victim to a cancer survivor.

It could have been done by someone else, but I selected him to fulfill this role for me. He also would be one of the very few men in my life who would see me with only one breast. He would see me "in the flesh," as they say. Only Dr. Yeo, my gynecologist, and my husband would have the opportunity to see me this way. As for the other men in my life, well, they would have to play the guessing game of "Which Boob Is It?"

Charlie's attitude and mannerisms about his feelings toward women's breasts would be very influential on me. If he treated them like they were insignificant, I might interpret that as all of me being insignificant. But if he made me feel that although they were important, they were not more important than my life, then I would have found someone who thought as I did, and as my husband did, and as my parents did.

I was blessed...he did exactly that. With the utmost professionalism, he explained to me that he knew losing my breast was a terrible thing. Having to be the surgeon to perform this unpleasant deed was equally awful. But knowing that my life would go on as a result of it made it the right thing to do. I had been in the presence of other surgeons when I was working as a clinical nurse, and had seen some who were caring and compassionate, and some who were cold and uncaring about what a patient who was losing a breast was going through.

I believe that surgeons have a very tough job when it comes to performing a mastectomy or any type of amputation. They have to be compassionate enough to empathize with the feelings of their patients, while simultaneously being objective and disconnected from the patient so they can perform the operation and keep their cool. Not all surgeons are made of the right stuff, and they don't all possess these qualities. No doubt Charlie's mother was proud of him. I knew that my mother would love him, too.

I remember the first time I'd been in an operating room as a young nurse. The first case I was to scrub in for was an above-the-knee amputation. The patient was in his mid-seventies and a brittle diabetic. Despite numerous hospitalizations, whirlpool baths, and removals of infected surface flesh, the man's leg continued to harbor a nasty infection that progressed into gas gangrene. The last option to save this man's life and prevent him from getting sepsis, which would result in death, was to remove his leg.

Because the man had a bad heart, the anesthesiologist felt he was at too great a risk to receive general anesthesia. Instead, he was given spinal anesthetic accompanied by hallucinogenic drugs. This meant that the patient would be technically awake but under the influence of powerful drugs during the operation. I was told that he would have absolutely no recall of it by that afternoon. When I came into the operating room that day, the patient was already on the table and surgery was about to start. Usually in an operating room things are fairly quiet. The only voices you hear are the surgeons asking for specific instruments to be passed to them. But this surgery was different, and as I said it was my first experience as a scrub nurse. The surgeon was an older man, brassy and tough, and he enjoyed giving student nurses a hard time. He was also a friend of my father's, so he took extra liberties with trying to joke with me and embarrass me whenever he could.

The procedure began. Instead of hearing only the voice of the surgeon, however, all we heard was the voice of the patient—he was singing! As the doctor proceeded to cut the skin, tie off various blood vessels, and expose the bone, the patient sang and sang. He didn't seem to realize he was in an operating room at all. But I knew I was, and this entire first experience completely unnerved me. Then the sawing began. The cutting of bone sounded and looked much like that of cutting a tree. Once the bone was cut through and the remaining flesh severed, the leg was no longer attached to the man's body. It was amazing to see this patient talking and singing while his leg was being completely disconnected from his body.

The surgeon looked at me and instructed me to pick up the limb and carry it to pathology down the hall. I was proud of myself that I had passed all the instruments he had asked for without dropping or fumbling even one of them. Now this? I was shaking. One of the

senior nursing staff attempted to intercede to complete this assignment for me, but the surgeon insisted that it was my job.

I took a deep breath and picked up the leg, holding it in my arms
by supporting it under the knee and ankle. I held it away from my
body. It felt warm and my stomach felt queasy. As I reached the
door of the O.R., the surgeon asked me to turn around so he could
"check something." He looked at the foot attached to the leg I was
holding and said, "Yep, that's what I thought. Look, Miss Dierker,
his toes are still wiggling."

I never got to look at those toes to verify what the surgeon had
just said. When I heard those words I fell onto the floor like a tree
being cut at its base. I fainted. All three legs hit the floor. When I
came to, lots of nurses were standing over me and the leg was gone.

One of the nurses said to me, "He shouldn't have done that to
you. He was getting nervous himself, and that was his way of
releasing tension. By refocusing everyone on you, he could forget
for a moment that he had made this patient a crippled man. This
gentleman has been a patient of his for years. It was very hard for
him to have to take his leg off, but it had to be done."

I was given the opportunity to scrub in for a lot of surgeries over
those next three months, but the first time was the only time I ever
fainted in the operating room. I looked at surgeons differently after
that experience. I was still angry that he had pulled a trick on me. (As
he said to me later, "Just lighten up, Miss Dierker. I was just pulling
your leg. I mean, making a joke. You take life too seriously.")

Well, I knew one thing. I didn't want to be in the operating room
with him for any mastectomies. No sir. And whenever a mastectomy was booked, I always took the other case that was scheduled
during the same block of time. Even though I knew I wouldn't be in
another situation where the patient was euphorically awake, I didn't
want to be asked to take someone's breast to the pathology department. I knew my stomach wouldn't be able to handle it. Nor would
my heart. I feared that I would relate the experience too much to that
of my friend, Miss Bertha. So I spared myself that experience.
Being with breast cancer patients in the recovery room and out in

the surgical nursing units tugged at my heartstrings enough. Soon there would be scrub nurses in the O.R. with me, and I would be the patient. I felt bad for them and hadn't even met them yet.

The day before my surgery I went to see Marla, my psychotherapist friend. She gave me a gift. It was a lovely compact of pressed powder with a mirror. She told me that she was giving it to me so I could see myself after the surgery and see what a breast cancer Survivors' face looked like.

She also told me that whenever she worried about her teenaged daughters, she pictured them being in protective bubbles of light. Inside these bubbles, no harm could come to them and they would remain safe, no matter what bad things were around them. She wanted me to picture myself in a special bubble of light that night and when I went into surgery in the morning. She gave me her private phone number and asked that Al call her as soon as I was out of surgery and back in my room fully recovered from anesthesia.

I picked up a videotape that a colleague, Earl Steinberg, had a friend of his Fed Ex to me at work. Earl was another key player in my adjustment to receiving my diagnosis, and also in helping me recover. The tape had been made by a breast surgeon at a major medical center in Boston. Still in its draft stages, the video was designed to show women diagnosed with breast cancer what the surgical scars look like. Its focus was on comparing lumpectomy surgery (also referred to as breast-sparing surgery) and mastectomy surgery. It showed photos of what reconstructive surgery results look like. The tape included interviews with women who represented each type of surgery. They talked of their feelings about the surgical options they had chosen.

Earl thought the tape would be of use to me. He, like I, knew that information equaled power and control. He didn't know how best to help me from a medical perspective, because this field of medicine was not his specialty. But he wanted to do whatever was in his power to provide me with the resources to get through this experience. I was very touched by his sincerity and compassion. Up until now, we had been primarily working colleagues, but this experience moved us to a higher plateau. I was thankful for his friendship.

Unfortunately, I lacked the nerve to watch the video before my own surgery. What if I heard somebody say that the absolutely best way to have this cancer removed was by a lumpectomy only? Could I possibly be influenced by the voice of an unknown person? What if someone on the tape said that women who don't have reconstruction right away would have suicidal tendencies? Would I believe such hogwash?

I had no idea what was on that tape. Though I believed it was probably a valuable reference for me, I elected not to watch it. I had made my decisions based on what I felt was the best medical advice I could possibly have received. I decided I would watch it after I was home and recovering from my surgery.

Al took me to Hunt Valley Mall that night in hopes of tiring me out by walking around and touring each of the stores. We were going to go to the movies, but that seemed like a waste of money. My mind would not have been on the show. We ran into two different people we knew and hadn't seen for a long time. These weren't friends per se, but acquaintances. Both people asked how we were and we responded with the patent answer "fine" and left it at that.

We left the mall around the time of its closing and drove home. My anxiety was building. I wondered if there was something I should be doing before I went to bed. Should there be some special ceremony to tell my breast good-bye? Should I take a picture? I decided that the answer was no. There was nothing to be done.

Dr. Beattie called me that night around ten as he said he would. I wanted to talk with him and hear him say one more time that the anesthesia would be no problem. He did. He was wonderful. He asked me to try to get a good night's sleep so that I would be ready for him in the morning. I told him I would try. After I hung up I turned on a cassette tape of some songs that my girlfriend Wanda and I had sung on my karaoke machine a few weeks before all this started. It was good to hear us singing, and even better to hear us laughing together. I wanted to hear us laughing again after tomorrow was behind me. I thought once again how we take life for granted. How we all too often don't realize just how precious each happy moment we have on this earth is. Al and I went to bed.

The time was 11:00. The house was quiet. Laura was staying with my mother-in-law for the night. We had received many phone calls all day and evening wishing me well and offering us prayers. Everything that could be done had been done to make tomorrow go well. The minute hand on the clock moved slowly that night. I was up and down walking around twice during the night. When I returned to bed the second time I was thinking about my grand mother Dierker, my father's mother. She had died several years ago and I still missed her. As I drifted off to sleep, I felt someone rubbing my leg. I sat up in bed but saw that no one was there. No one I could see, anyway. Al was asleep. I believe my grandmother was there in the bedroom with me that night, letting me know I'd be okay. That this would all turn out okay.

Eventually the alarm clock went off at 4:45 a.m. I arose, took a shower, and got dressed. The house was extremely quiet. Neither Al nor I were talking. Just silent gestures of hugs as we passed each other in the hall. I decided to wear comfortable clothes, so I dressed in my favorite blue shirt and a pair of shorts. Certainly not the usual attire I wore to work, but this day I wasn't going to the hospital as an employee, I was going as a patient.

We arrived at the hospital around 5:45 a.m. and I was due to report to the presurgical area at 6:00 a.m. Al dropped me off at the entrance so I could use the bathroom. My stomach was grumbling and I knew that I would have the green-apple-quick-steps before I got to the Same Day Surgery area.

As I entered the hospital at this ungodly hour, I spotted someone I was very pleased to see. It was our hospital chaplain, Clyde Shallenberger. He walked over to me and inquired about what I was doing there at this very early hour, and why I was dressed funny. I took his hands and told him of my situation. He hugged me and said that he'd be by to see me after surgery, and that while I was in the O.R. he'd pray for me (or, as he sometimes says, "talk with the boss"). I felt very much at peace having run into him like that. I still have absolutely no idea what Clyde was doing there at that hour, but I was certainly glad to see him. Perhaps the hour wasn't as ungodly as I had thought.

Al joined me just a few minutes later, and we held hands as we took the elevator up to the fifth floor. Six families were already waiting outside the pre-op area for the doors to be unlocked. Soon a nurse came, letting us all inside en masse. One by one the receptionist called our names, and one by one each patient was identified from the group that he or she was seated with.

Soon my name was called and I was given some forms to fill out. As I completed them, my eyes kept drifting up. I watched two parents sitting with their small child. The child was about three and mentally retarded. The two parents had the patience of saints. Apparently the child was the patient and couldn't have anything to eat or drink. He would point to his mouth and cry. His mother picked him up and told him he wasn't allowed to have anything, and that she was sorry. He'd cry. Then she'd pull out some toys from a large bag she had brought with her.

One of the toys was a music box. She wound it up and gave it to him. He instantly stopped crying and held the box right up against his ear. He sat there on the floor and rocked himself, holding the music box near his face.

I looked at this family and realized how truly blessed I was. My child was normal. My family was healthy. And after this ordeal today, I, too, would once again be a well person, I hoped.

After a few moments went by, my name was called and I was escorted into an exam room. Al was allowed to come with me. I was asked to remove my clothes and put on a hospital gown, hat, and booties. "We'll be wheeling you into the operating room from here, Mrs. Shockney, so you'll need to say good-bye to your husband now."

Al leaned down and kissed me twice. "I love you. I'll see you soon." Tears began to flow down my cheeks. I prayed to God not to let me make a fool of myself when I reached the operating room.

I had this terrible fear that I would lose my cool and turn into a screaming bantam chicken, pleading with the doctor not to proceed with the operation.

In a matter of moments I was at the door of the operating room. I could hear the scrub nurses talking and the sounds of the stainless steel portable carts being wheeled into place. I was so glad that my contact lenses were out so the room was unfocused. I didn't want to see any scalpels or other instruments. I was asked to stand and position myself on the operating room table. My heart was racing.

Dr. Beattie came in and looked down at me. "Well, Lillie, how much sleep did you get for me last night?" I told him I had gotten the same amount that I had gotten when I was in hard labor with my daughter at the time of her birth. He patted my hand. I got a grip on him and couldn't let go. He reassured me that all would go well. A resident was with him and he introduced himself to me. His eyes were kind. He had the assignment of putting the IV in my hand.

Dr. Beattie then told me he'd be giving me a drug called madazalam to make me feel good, and that I'd forget my troubles within a few seconds of its being injected through my IV. When he injected the medicine it burned. He tried to cheer me up and lighten my emotional load by telling me that this medicine would make me tell all of the Hopkins' hospital secrets I knew. It was an effective distraction. I was suddenly no longer focused on my breast, but instead worried that I might tell tales out of school.

When I closed my eyes, I heard my mother singing in my head. She was singing a song I used to enjoy hearing her sing by special request at the churches she frequented. It was called "He Gazed Up and Smiled on Me." It was a religious song about a person meeting Christ along the side of the road. I felt perfectly calm now. I was here for a good reason, not a bad one. I was here to be transformed from a breast cancer victim to a breast cancer survivor. That was what I wanted. And with that, I fell asleep.

Chapter 12

The next voice I heard was Dr. Beattie's telling me that I was in the recovery room and that my surgery was over. I had trouble opening my eyes but could hear his voice plainly. I remember asking him if I had told any Hopkins' secrets, and he reassured me that I hadn't. I believed him, but not completely. For all I knew, the surgical team had set up a microphone near my head so that any politically hot secrets I might have blabbed could be electronically recorded. I definitely wanted to get the next publication of the *Hopkins Hotline* to make sure there wasn't a one-page spread dedicated to me entitled "Director of Q.A. Tells All While Under the Influence of Drugs."

I wanted to move my hands up to my chest but initially lacked the strength to do so. Eventually I was able to slide both of my hands up. I placed one hand over each breast area. I felt nothing on either side! Just flatness. Flat as a pancake. I called out for a nurse. Any nurse. A young woman dressed in scrubs hastened over to me. "Are you in pain, Mrs. Shockney?"

I told her no. I wanted to know what had been done to me. I couldn't feel either breast. What had happened? Had someone made a mistake and taken off the wrong one, then after discovering the error removed the one we knew did have cancer? Or did the doctor get more information from the pathology department that made him biopsy the right breast and subsequently discover that it, too, was cancerous?

No, none of these fears was true. The nurse explained that my left breast was gone and that I had on a very tight binder which compressed the dressings to prevent swelling. Because the binder went all the way around me, that was why my right breast seemed to not be there either. What a relief! But as I mentally concentrated on feeling the sensation of my right breast (the remaining one), I realized that I felt as if my left breast were there, too. I asked the question again of the recovery room nurse.

"Tell me just what, exactly, was done. Did Charlie do the mastectomy as planned?" She answered yes again. She then checked the hemovacs. I could see each of the drainage containers when she held them up to look at the amount of bloody fluid in them.

Still woozy from the effects of the anesthesia, I looked around the room as best I could. Many stretchers with patients on them were visible and lots of moaning could be heard. My mind drifted back to my nursing experiences with recovery room patients. When they awakened they were often confused as to where they were. Their faces grimaced with signs of pain.

Beside me on the stretcher to my left I heard a woman moaning and yelling out. "Is it gone? Oh no, it is. God help me." A nurse came over to her and took her hand. The patient didn't speak any more—she just cried. The nurse didn't speak either. She simply held the patient's hand and stroked her forehead. The woman soon drifted back to sleep. I called the nurse over to me. "Is she okay? She sounded so upset." The nurse responded and her words came as no surprise to me. It was what I had surmised. I was lying beside a newly enlisted club member like myself. She, too, had a mastectomy. Her left breast was gone, just like mine. I wanted to turn over and look at her, but my lack of strength prevented me from doing so. Soon she was taken away to the nursing unit where she would complete her recovery.

Complete her recovery—that really wasn't correct. Neither of us was going to complete our recovery here at the hospital. Soon, we would be well enough to go home, but the majority of our recovery would take place far from these walls. I wanted to start working on those steps to recovery as soon as I could. My transformation was complete and it was time to focus my attention on getting well and getting on with my life. I never got to meet the other patient who had her transformation surgery done simultaneously with mine. I hope she did well and has been blessed with the necessary support systems it takes to get through the post-surgical steps to recovery.

My husband was allowed to come into the recovery room to be with me. I was told at a later time that I had been calling out for him. I don't remember doing this, but patients often do things in the recovery room that they erase from their minds instantaneously. Al was all smiles, with only a few hives on his face. When Al is under stress, he gets hives. He looks as if someone took red lifesavers and stuck them all over his face. That's the only place he ever gets hives. It is always easy to see just how high his stress level is by the number of red lifesavers I can count on his face.

I remember when we bought our house and went to settlement, he had about fourteen hives on his face. He was truly a lumpy, bumpy mess. He'd had only a few bumps until he saw how much money we would be paying for our home by the time it was paid off in thirty years. Seeing that dollar figure surely did it to him. The hives appeared rapidly. By the time he read the numbers and signed his name, they were all over his face and neck.

Looking at him standing at the foot of my stretcher with all those lumps and bumps on his face made me worry that he knew something about how the surgery went that I didn't know. He reassured me that everything had gone fine, and that Dr. Yeo had spoken to him and to my parents and gave all of them a good report on me. Al's hives were from worrying that I'd have trouble with the anesthesia. But he had been reassured by Dr. Beattie that all was well with that, too. He looked very happy and just couldn't stop smiling at me and telling me that he loved me. Various nurses came over to him and told him I was doing well. He just beamed all the more.

Patients say funny things sometimes. This time I was the one being funny, rather than being the nurse who got to hear the funny comments. Al told me I kept telling everyone in the recovery room that I felt as if something was standing on the left side of my chest. Apparently upon inquiry, I further explained to those within earshot that an elephant was standing on my chest. When Al asked me about the elephant, I assured him it was only a little elephant, just a baby, and that it was okay for it to be there. Who knows, maybe I thought I was Dumbo's mother.

Eventually I was stable enough to be moved to my room in the nursing unit, and Al left me temporarily to make arrangements for the phone to be connected in my room. As I traveled down the hallway, my stomach felt queasy and I was relieved to finally be in a bed where I could position the head of my bed a little higher.

Soon Al returned. Right behind him were my parents. Dad stood at the side of my bed. I said hello as if greeting people for a gathering of sorts. Dad was tearful. Mom looked relieved but very tired. Her five weeks of worrying were plainly visible on her face. Dad didn't want to stay, but I insisted that they not rush off so quickly. I think he was afraid he would get too emotional and not project the image of a tough guy. But he had been a tough guy in my book. A tough guy for me was someone who is strong when the going gets tough. And let's face it, the going had gotten pretty tough for all of us.

Mom and Dad kissed me. Each told me they loved me. Mom said she'd see me the next day when Al brought me home. I wondered what was racing through their minds after all of these weeks of anguish and torture. Being parents is truly a lifetime job that requires you to be on call twenty-four hours a day. Surely they would both get good check marks in God's giant book for enduring this experience.

Right before Mom and Dad left, Al pulled a note out of his pocket that Laura had given him. She had asked that it be given to me as soon as I was back in my room. It was sealed in an envelope; it obviously contained highly confidential material and was for my eyes only. I had Al open the envelope for me, and then I took the paper out and read it aloud. It was a poem. It was dated July 9, 1992, so I knew she had written it five days before. It was appropriately entitled "Appearance."

Appearance

Nobody's perfect
Just look at me
But if you really think about it
Who wants to be.

Beauty and glamour
Are nice to get
But it's what inside that counts
You must never forget.

I hope you understand
What I've been trying to say
I hope you get well soon
And I love you more and more each day.

Love,
Laura

When your child who is all of twelve writes something philosophically marvelous, it's hard to keep a dry eye in the room. As you can imagine, there were no dry eyes in my hospital room that afternoon. I thought it wonderful that someone so young would be so wise. Children usually adjust so well to crisis situations. They are so resilient. At what age do we lose this wonderful way to view the world?

I once again hoped and prayed that her analytical approach to dealing with this family crisis would never be tested when she became an adult herself. Oh please, God, don't let this ever happen to my baby. She is too special to have to be confronted with such an unpleasant and evil thing as breast cancer.

I glanced up at my mother's face and understood, at least a little bit, just how devastating this experience must have been for her—and still was for her. It seemed as if she was aging with worry right before my eyes.

As a matter of fact, a few nights before my surgery, my grand-mother had called me to talk for a while. She was worrying about my mother and how much older she appeared to have become in only a matter of weeks. She said, "She is worrying so, I know that you are going to be all right. She needs to sleep more and worry less. I think the wrinkles in her face are so bad now that even Oil of Olay isn't going to help."

Just think of it, four generations of women. And three out of four of them worrying about her daughter. It was amazing to think about it and even more amazing to be experiencing it.

My folks left shortly after I read Laura's poem. I hoped that tonight they would each worry a little bit less.

Soon I started having visitors. First Diane, Scott, and Marge came by. They looked relieved to see me and glad that my surgery was over. They didn't stay long so they would not exhaust me. I appreciated their consideration about my fatigue level. They also ran interference for me to prevent an entourage of people from coming to my door. Though everyone meant well, having continu-ous visitation was not in my best interests at the time. They knew that, and encouraged others to recognize it as well. They carried status reports back to my staff and other hospital employees who were anxious to know how things had gone.

Earl came by for a visit that evening. Such a dear man. I knew that he had an unbearable schedule, but despite it, before he went home he came by to see how I was doing. Tim also came by. So did Clyde, the hospital chaplain. I told Clyde that "his boss" had done a good job and had obviously responded to the many requests (prayers) that had been submitted to him by various and sundry people on my behalf. Clyde smiled and held my hand for a moment, then departed.

My stomach started misbehaving about that time, and before long I was throwing up. I threw up every ten to fifteen minutes from 4:00 p.m. until 8:30 p.m. Al patiently held the emesis basin as I'd give one more heave. Eventually the anti-nausea medicine took effect and my stomach quieted down. I was offered pain medicine several times, but did not feel the need to take it. Usually painkillers upset my stomach, and I had done all the throwing up I intended to do. There was no sense in taking something that I knew would only make me end up with my head in the trash can again.

Al left late that night. I didn't want him to go, but he had to pick up Laura from his mother's and I knew that my daughter needed time with him, too. He had called everyone on our list of contacts to let them know that I was out of surgery and doing reasonably well. He was operating from nervous energy that day. He kissed me and held my hand. It was a special night for us to share together.

A resident came in to see me from the surgical team shortly after Al left. He checked my bandages, which required him to unfasten my binder. I held my breath when he did this. I was afraid of feeling pain, but even more frightened that my eyes would be tempted to glance downward and look at the surgical site. It was no trouble resisting this temptation, though.

He told me that he had been in the operating room with me that day. Though I believed Dr. Beattie's telling me that I hadn't told any stories out of school, I was curious if I had said anything after I was under the effects of the drugs. The resident told me that I had made one request before I was completely under. That request was to be "reassembled" in the event that something went wrong and I didn't wake up.

I must have thought that I was like the character Number 5 in the movie *Short Circuit*. For those of you who haven't seen the movie, Number 5 was a computerized robot with artificial intelligence. At least the scientists who created the robot thought he was artificial. Later they discovered that he had somehow taken on human qualities and could think on his own and feel emotion. In part of the movie, strategic plans were being made to capture and disassemble him. When Number 5 overheard the scientists discussing their plans he said, "Disassemble?! NO disassemble!!"

I found it curious that I would make such a similar "last request." I guess my subconscious didn't want to give up my breast

if it wasn't absolutely necessary. And if I were to die on the operating table, there certainly would be no good reason why it
shouldn't be reattached and buried with me.

I recalled having told a girlfriend of mine that if I had opted to
have reconstruction done and died on the operating room table
from an anesthesia complication, I would want to be laid out in my
casket nude from the waist up. I'd want everyone to see just what
I had died for. Heck, such a death would have seemed completely
senseless to me if your friends didn't get to see what you were willing to sacrifice your life for. They could say, "Well, would you look
at the bodacious tah-tahs on Lillie. She wasn't ever really happy
with having to settle for only one...one tah. Well, she didn't get to
see the newly created one, but she sure would have been pleased
with it."

When the resident told me about my last request, I realized just
how frightened I had really been about being put to sleep. Who
could blame me, though? I had a pretty crappy track record with
anesthetic agents.

At approximately 9:30 p.m. a strange woman entered my room
carrying a large plastic bag and her purse. She came over and introduced herself as Eileen. She was a Reach to Recovery volunteer. I
was surprised to see her there so late but welcomed the opportunity to visit with her. She sat at my bedside and spoke very softly. As
she spoke she began slowly removing objects from her plastic bag.
First she pulled out a small, pink cotton rectangular pillow and
offered to place it under my left elbow. She said that these pillows
were made by recovered breast cancer patients and were designed
to provide a little extra support for my affected arm. Next she took
out some reading material that contained information about places
to buy a prosthesis, mastectomy bras, wigs for patients who might
be going through chemotherapy, and a list of support groups in the
immediate area.

She asked me about my experience with breast cancer thus far.
Things such as how was I diagnosed, had I planned on reconstruction, did the doctor anticipate chemotherapy, and so on. Next she

took out a bra that appeared to be something like a sports bra but much stretchier and softer. She explained that when the doctor gave me the go-ahead to come out of my binder and the hemovacs were removed, I would be able to wear this as a bra until I was ready to be fitted for a breast prosthesis. Usually most surgeons prefer that the patient be six to seven weeks post-op before they go for a fitting. That way the fitting can be done correctly and without interference from chest and arm edema.

She then took out a bag of cotton batting, the kind one would stuff a pillow with. She began tearing off small pieces and putting them in the left pocket of this soft, stretchy bra. I asked her what she was doing. I wasn't prepared for the answer. She said she was making a temporary breast prosthesis for me out of the cotton. I stared at this woman's hands as she tore off another swatch of cotton batting and slowly pushed it into the bra pocket. Then I lost it. I started crying and asked her to stop. "Please don't do that. I can't lie here in this bed and watch you tearing off the cotton like that." My breast was only a wad of cotton batting.

I felt completely helpless and demoralized. Perhaps if she had come in the room with the cotton batting already in the bra it wouldn't have been so bad, but watching her manually assemble a supposed breast out of that cotton made me ill.

She graciously gathered up the cotton and put it and the bra back in the bag and placed it at the foot of my bed. She told me that it was my option to wear a prosthesis or not. (She was a very tiny woman, and I would say was not wearing any prosthesis; she'd had bilateral mastectomies.) I think that a woman who normally wore a 42D bra would look pretty silly without a prosthesis. But I chose to reserve those comments. She had meant well in her visit to me. She had come as a volunteer and I appreciated her doing so. She left shortly after.

Once the volunteer left, the room was quiet and visitor-free for the first time all day. I felt a little uncomfortable being alone. I didn't want to be there without anyone. I think I was afraid if left alone I'd have too much time to really think and reflect about the events of the day. My mind was overwhelmed as it was, and I didn't want to think any more, not right now. Thank heavens the door to my room opened once again and Jean came in.

Jean was the breast cancer nurse specialist. She was working very late that day and swung by to see how I was doing. She checked my dressings and told me that Dr. Yeo (Charlie) would come by in the morning to review with me his discharge instructions and how he wanted me to record my hemovac drainage. I told her that Al would also be in early in the morning but that the person who'd be helping me with the dressings would be my mother. I would be able to show her what needed to be done.

I told Jean that I wasn't ready for Al to look at my incision yet, and she said that was okay. Shortly thereafter she left my room. I was impressed that she had taken the time to come by to see me, particularly because of the lateness of the hour.

It was now approaching 11:00 p.m., the time for nurses to change shifts. Myck, a very attractive Asian nurse, poked her head in to see me one last time before she went out to make her report at the end of her shift. She came over to my bedside to check the amount of fluid left in my IV bag. Just as she prepared to leave I started to cry. I don't know exactly what I was crying about. There were so many reasons to cry that I'm not sure I singled out any particular one to initiate the flood that rolled down my face.

Despite the fact that the evening shift report was due, that more patients' IVs needed to be checked, and other duties needed attending to, Myck did what I used to pride myself on doing when I had worked bedside as a clinical nurse. Myck sat down on my bed and took my hand. She just sat. No words, no glancing at her watch because her shift was over. She waited for me to speak. I think she would have waited with me all night had I not spoken and expressed what was on my mind.

I said, "I've taken care of many patients in my life. Many patients who have gone through what I have just experienced. I've sat on the bed with these patients, as you are now with me, and held their hands and cried with them. I never once imagined that some day someone would be sitting in a white uniform with me."

Tears ran down Myck's face now, too. She didn't speak. We embraced. I reassured her that I would be all right and asked that she finish her rounds and give her report. She stood by my bed for a moment longer, squeezed my hand, and wished me well. Then she departed.

That was one of the longest nights of my life. I slept very little. Each time I awakened, I had to get myself reoriented as to where I was and why I was there. My recovery from this ordeal would definitely require more than a bathtub full of Calgon bubbles. Oh Calgon, take me away...

Chapter 13

I watched the sunrise through my hospital room window. The nursing unit was just starting its morning activity. I could hear the nursing staff talking in the hall and the sound of stretcher wheels as the night shift completed its final activities of the early morning, which consisted primarily of prepping patients who were having surgery that morning.

Soon my door swung open and Al walked through. What a welcome sight he was! He kissed me and asked me how my night had been. Just as he sat down beside me, the day shift nurse came in and removed the IV from my hand. She told us that the surgical team would soon be in to change my bandages before I went home. She also said that she would be back shortly after breakfast to show Al how to empty my hemovac drainage bags.

"I don't want you in the room when the surgeons come in to change my dressings," I said firmly to Al. "Your job will be to manage the hemovacs. Mom and I will worry about the bandages. Deal?" He nodded in agreement and I felt relieved.

Since I hadn't been very successful in keeping a lot of food down because of the anesthesia, I had only liquids for breakfast. They slid down easily, thank goodness. Just as I finished, the nurse came back and started her instructions regarding the drains. They had to be emptied four times a day and the amount of drainage measured and recorded on a paper she gave us. She showed Al how she emptied the drain labeled #1, and then he emptied the #2 drain under her supervision. He did fine. Nervous, but fine.

The nurse had just left the room when the door swung open again and there standing before us was Charlie Yeo.

He was chipper, dressed in scrubs and his long white coat. He swiftly walked over to me and before I could answer his question of how my night had been, he maneuvered himself into a sitting position beside me on the bed and unfastened my binder.

I was petrified. This was happening so fast. Before I could even prepare for my defense, he asked Al to come over and help him change my dressing. My heart was racing and my palms sweating. I was unable to speak. I wanted to yell out, "Hey. Wait just a cotton-pickin' minute. This isn't the deal. I don't want my husband to see my incision yet!" But I was unable to get my lips to move.

As Charlie removed all of the bandages, I could feel the coolness of the air on my chest. My eyes were fixed on Al's face. I was watching his every move, every blink, waiting to see a look of disgust, a look of rejection. I saw only a look of seriousness. He wanted to make sure that the way he was putting the new bandages on the wound met with the physician's approval.

I don't think I could have felt any worse if a team of doctors had come in my room, stood me naked on my head, spread my legs, and used a protoscope to look up my rear end while video projected the entire procedure onto a fifty-inch TV screen set up in the main corridor of the hospital for all to see.

It was awful. But when it was over, Al looked up at me and said, "It looks fine. We're going to be fine." I knew then that Charlie had done perhaps one of the best things he ever could have done for me, for us. By showing Al how he wanted the dressings changed each day, he had also shown me that we were going to be okay. My scar was not going to be a barrier to our maintenance of a good relationship and marriage.

I don't know if Charlie does this with all the husbands or if he sizes up the situation and makes that judgment call as the circumstances allow. He is a clever man. For all I know, he and Al had planned the whole thing. It doesn't matter now. It's in the past. But it was a moment I will always remember. (I'm still annoyed that I didn't get to see Al without his teeth. I was cheated out of that Kodak moment.)

Scott and Diane came up to the room just as we were preparing to leave. Their timing was perfect. This gave Al the opportunity to go downstairs, get the car, and bring it around to the front entrance while my two special friends escorted me out of the hospital in a wheelchair.

I wore the shorts I had worn to the hospital and a large (better described as jumbo) button-up-the-front shirt that I had purchased especially for this day. It was a size forty-eight. (See, I said it was jumbo.) Because my hair gets very oily at night and it wasn't washed that morning, I wore a hat and my glasses. Even if an employee who knew me well had seen me, I doubted he or she would have recognized me. As a matter of fact, quite a few people I knew were in the hallway and walked right by me. I was very relieved about that.

Soon I was out at the car and tucked safely into the front seat for the ride home. Scott, Diane, and I must have looked like we were saying good-bye for a decade. Everyone's eyes were damp.

Once we reached home, Mom came out to the car to help us get all our gear into the house. She still looked as if she had gotten little sleep, and it was clear that her migraine headaches had persisted. I felt very awkward walking around with the drainage hoses safely pinned to my shirt. I had this constant fear that the pin would pop and the drains would rip right out of my chest cavity. Even though I knew this couldn't happen (because they were actually sutured in), I worried about it constantly. I told people that the hemovacs felt like hand grenades. If I made the wrong move they'd go POW!

Laura was glad to see me. She came over and gave me a kiss. Because of her weak stomach, she never stayed in my room long. If she had lingered, I think the sight of the hand grenades would have caused her to throw up. She did say, "See, you said that you would look different, but you don't to me. Other than wearing your glasses instead of your contact lenses you look just the same."

I told her that I looked different under my clothes. She was unimpressed with this statement. She simply replied that no one could see me under there "so it doesn't count."

Mom helped me change into a nightgown. I had purchased three "one size fits all." (The manufacturers had wised up and the tags actually read, "one size fits most.") These gowns were smart investments for me. They slipped easily over my head, had a very large head opening and scooped-out neckline, and were very full and flowing. There was ample room for me and my surgical army weapons.

We were home only about twenty minutes when the doorbell rang. The local florist was delivering a gorgeous bouquet of flowers. The doorbell rang a lot that week. With the flowers and balloons alone, I received more than twenty get-well wishes. I also received other special treasures, like a stuffed cow, whimsical cow pin, cow eggs, stuffed bunnies, baskets, fragranced soap, books, and other lovely gifts. Each was from someone very special to me. (See Chapter 21 for a list of recommended gifts for a club member you might know.) Being surrounded by so many lovely bouquets of flowers and other well-wishing memorabilia was very uplifting. The messages on the gift cards were also special, and I kept every one. I also took pictures of the floral arrangements. To receive so many exquisite bouquets you usually have to be dead. How fortunate I was to receive them and personally get to enjoy them.

My first night home was a restless one. Al decided I should have the bed to myself, so he slept downstairs on the sofa. Mom slept in Laura's room.

I love pillows. To tell you the truth, I have so many pillows on our bed that a friend of ours calls our house "the House of Pillows." Four standard-sized pillows stay on our bed; three of them for me. Two go under my head and one between my knees. Because I needed to support my left arm—my surgical side—one more pillow was added to this pile. My husband has learned over our fifteen years together that once a pillow gets added to the bed it never leaves. I also kept in bed with me my little pink pillow made by the Reach to Recovery volunteers. It made me feel close to club members even though none were physically there.

The next morning Al and Mom helped me get up and moving. By now I had gone two and a half days without washing my hair and that distressed me. I wasn't able to do anything about it, though.

Get well cards started coming in. The phone rang often, too. Each card that arrived I read with great care. I saved them all. In less than two weeks' time more than two hundred cards were delivered to our mailbox. I was amazed by how much I was cared about and loved.

Cards are very special to me. I love sending cards. For that matter, I love reading cards. I can stand in a card store for several hours and laugh my head off reading humorous cards. I'm the one you see in the store who becomes so hysterical with laughter that I feel compelled to share the humorous moment, and walk up to a total stranger to show her the card I just read. Sometimes people laugh with me; other times they just stare at me and walk away. Oh well, their loss.

Below are just a few of my favorite verses from the get well wishes I received. Unfortunately, I can't show you the accompanying picture on the front of each card, but trust me, each was perfect for its verse.

Remember, when you're feeling so low you have to reach up to touch bottom...whose bottom it is can make a big difference!

I know things look tough right now. But hang in there. Otherwise I'll be forced to call you and sing, "High Hopes" really loud and off key.

Some days it's tougher to hang in there than others. Like the days you wear a really old bra with worn elastic.

Sometimes a friendly little smile can make your day...but usually it takes money or sex.

Wouldn't it be nice if our lives were like VCRs...and we could "fast forward" through the crummy times?

Relax. Things could be worse. You could be stuck in a hot

elevator with a bunch of gross guys who went to an all-you-can-eat burrito buffet for lunch.

Aw, c'mon! Cuddly-Wuddly Bear wants you to cheer up! Kinda makes you wanna squeeze Cuddly-Wuddly Bear's little neck until his itsy-witsy button eyes pop off, doesn't it.

Remember: You're not fully dressed without a smile...Oh, and underpants.

It's awfully hard to feel bad when you open a card that says something that tickles your funny bone just right. I also received a lot of lively inspirational cards. Cards that focused on the value of friendship, family, religion. All of these cards are kept in a wooden basket that Diane brought me as a gift. I still look through them periodically and read the messages written to me by so many dear friends.

Mom and Al got things down to a science when it came to fixing meals, answering the phone, opening mail, and helping me get around the house. All in all, we were managing fairly well in the Shockney household. Don't get me wrong—a lot of tears were shed, but there was also a lot of laughter.

One of the funniest moments came on my third day home. I couldn't stand my hair glued to my scalp any longer and decided that it was time for a shampoo. I couldn't get in the shower because of my bandages, neither could I lean over the sink. It was a dilemma, but one I was determined to solve. Improvisation became the name of the game. While Al was outside getting the newspaper and Mom was in Laura's room getting dressed, I grabbed a Hefty trash bag from the kitchen and proceeded to cut a hole in it for my head. When Al and Mom next saw me, I was shrouded up in a dark green Hefty bag with just my head sticking out. "Come! We're all going to wash my hair!" Into the shower we all went. We put a folding chair in the shower stall and Al held the shower head in his hands. I bent over as far as I could and Mom kept towels around my neck in case of leakage around the opening in the bag.

Al said to me, "Well, don't you look like a prize right now...wrapped up in a Hefty bag like an escaped lunatic." I told him that I was a prize, a booby prize. It was at that moment I renamed my hemovac drainage bags booby traps! We laughed a lot that morning.

I felt great after my hair was washed. I looked better, too. Each morning until I gained shower privileges, I got my hair washed using the Hefty bag system. I definitely looked like a modern art version of a bag lady.

By Friday, just four days after my mastectomy, the drainage had dramatically subsided. I had my first appointment with Charlie that morning. He would check my hemovacs and decide if they could be removed. I wanted the booby traps gone, but I was afraid of having them yanked out.

Charlie saw me within five minutes of my arrival. He took me in the exam room and requested that my family wait in the reception area. He unveiled the incision and read the record that we had meticulously kept of the drainage amounts from each container. He decided that the drainage was decreased enough and it was okay to pull both drains. Usually he kept one of the drains in for seven days, but he was going out of town and felt that my risk of developing a seroma (a pocket of fluid that can form along the incision or in the axillary area) was minimal. He had me lie on the exam table and asked me to hold onto the railings of the table while he pulled the first hose out. He said, "Now keep your hands on the side rails and don't move them. I'm afraid that if you move them, you'll locate them up to my throat." With that he pulled the first hose. It took only a second. My chest vibrated as he removed a hose that was equal in length to a garden snake. Then he pulled the second one out. I was finally free of those crazy contraptions and felt one step closer to recovery.

Charlie was pleased with my healing thus far. I told him that I had my father's skin, which usually healed well with just a fine line of a scar. He asked me how things were going, and I told him "okay." When he asked if I had looked at the incision yet, I told him "no." He didn't press the issue.

I also told him about my phantom limb sensation and phantom limb pain. He seemed intrigued with this. I told him that the evening before I was sitting at the kitchen table for dinner and suddenly felt as if someone were gently biting my nipple—the nipple that was no longer there. I told him it seemed so weird to me. I didn't know what to say to my family about it. My mother knew that something wasn't quite right with me by the expression on my face. I elected not to say anything, but I felt embarrassed, so I got up from the table and went into the bathroom until the feeling went away.

Charlie smiled at me and said, "I bet you didn't tell your mother." He was right!

My mother went home that Friday afternoon. She had stayed through the worst of my recovery period and was ready to head back home to the farm where Dad had been fending for himself. That was never a required skill for him to learn. He has the basics down, like making coffee and zapping a hot dog in the microwave, but beyond that he isn't much of a chef. When Mom had been away from him in the past, she usually prepared a turkey, a ham, and a roast. (Please note that I said, "and," not "or.") Dad is a big eater. When Mom isn't around, I think his nervous system must activate his stomach into thinking that it is hungry when it isn't.

Dad is also a big lover of chocolate candy. When Mom is away, Dad is known to gain weight from all of the sweets and entrees she leaves for him. Actually, Mom doesn't leave him candy; he provides that for himself. In fact, when Mom does buy candy she usually hides it.

One time she hid some chocolate in the freezer underneath the green beans, thinking he would never find it. On a day that Laura and I were visiting, he went to the utility room to get something out of the freezer and returned looking like a Cheshire cat. He was holding a Hershey bar in his hand and saying, "Mom thinks that I can't smell chocolate when it's frozen, but she's wrong." He had actually found Mom's stash several days before and had nearly depleted it by the time Mom discovered that her hiding place had been found.

While Mom was helping to take care of me, there was no doubt in my mind that Dad was eating a lot of sweets and treats. It was best that she head home to get him back on a balanced diet again.

The following morning I decided it was time for me to look at my incision. I had Al hold up a mirror while I unfastened the binder and peeled off the bandages. Despite my having cared for other mastectomy patients and having already seen the effects of the surgery, I found that my own incision shocked me. I had pictured it in my mind many times, but seeing it for real was overwhelming. Tears silently streamed down my face.

Al reassured me by saying he thought it looked okay. I just kept shaking my head no and continuing to look in the mirror. It was really gone. Even though it felt like it was still there, it wasn't. There was nothing there now but a long scar signifying that something was gone. I had to concentrate on why it wasn't there. The flesh that had been there had cancer in it, and if left to its own devices would have killed me. In exchange for God sparing me and my family the loss of my life, I had lost a breast. I realized this was a very fair exchange, but one that would require more mental adjustment. In time, it would be okay.

About ten days after my surgery, I was granted the privilege of removing the binder and keeping it off. No seromas had formed, which I was quite pleased about. I was now able to wear the bra that the Reach to Recovery volunteer had brought me. I took it out of the bag and looked at it. I felt the cotton batting she had placed inside the left pocket of the bra cup. My girlish figure had been traded in for stuff and fluff. It certainly didn't feel like a breast, but it would have to serve as a substitute until the artificial breast prosthesis was obtained. I added some more cotton batting and tried it on. I took it off again and tried to adjust the shape of the cotton in the cup of the bra so it looked something like a breast.

Before I put the bra back on, I glanced down at my feet. Good grief! I could see my feet! I had not been able to look down and see my feet since age fourteen! My left foot was in plain view, and because of my remaining right breast I had a partial view of my right foot. I found this amazing. I went into the bathroom and decided to clip my toenails. Suddenly what had always been an awkward task became simple. I could see my toes and reach for them without my boobs being in the way. So this is how a man cuts his toenails. Boy, do they have it easy!

I returned to the bedroom and put on my soft stuff-and-fluff bra. I looked in the mirror. Not a bad disguise, I thought, considering what it's made of. I put on a loosely fitting shirt. Al was impressed with the illusion. Yeah, this would serve as an acceptable disguise until better provisions could be made. It was funny. I found myself forgetting, if only for a few seconds, that my breast was gone. I was on the road to recovery for sure now. Yes, there would be more bumps in the road ahead, but I felt thankful for and proud of the progress I had made so far.

Chapter 14

I felt well enough to start taking short rides in the car with Al and Laura. Trips to the store for ice cream. Quick jaunts to the bank. I still seemed to lack the energy for long outings. I also worried that people around me would bump into me and hurt my chest.

There were times I felt like making a sign to wear on my chest that said, "Danger. Standing too close to this object could be dangerous to your health." I thought this would be an appropriate sign because I knew if anyone bumped me and hurt my incision I would deck them for sure. Perhaps a different sign would be self-explanatory: "This may appear to be a boob, but it isn't. Getting too close to it could jeopardize your personal safety."

I worried that strangers would notice that this was not a real breast but merely stuff and fluff. Let's face it. It didn't bounce. Not only that, but the left side of the bra had a tendency to ride up because there was no weight in it to hold it down. I experimented by putting quarters in it to help give it a little weight, but it rode up on my chest anyway. I felt as if people were looking at me and wondering why one breast was two inches higher than the other. It seemed as if I was constantly asking Al if my boobs were "lined up all right."

When you get right down to it, I doubt anyone was looking at my chest at all, but you wouldn't have been able to convince me of that at the time.

By my third week of recovery, I started having work brought to me from the hospital. Several employees who work for me alternated making deliveries and picking up completed work on a daily basis. Though my energy level was still low, it made me feel good to be productive and back in a semi-working environment. It was also good to have visits from my staff. Marge became a regular visitor, and she, Diane, and Scott would leave funny notes for me in my folders that would keep me laughing when I really felt like crying.

One afternoon, Al and his brother, Jack, decided to take me to the movies. This was to be my first venture out for more than a quick pit stop. The three of us went to see *Death Becomes Her*. It was great! Right up my alley! Black humor at its best!

Here were two women about my age who would do anything to ensure that their bodies remained looking like that of a voluptuous twenty-one-year-old. They paid an extraordinary amount of money to receive a potion that guaranteed them youth for an eternity. Of course, there was a catch to this marvelous miracle. They would live forever, as well, but they had to be very careful with their bodies. If they broke an arm, it could not be repaired in the usual and conventional ways, with plaster of Paris. No, their bodies required crazy glue and lots of spray paint, and in what better color than "#9 flesh tone."

In the movie, their wrinkles magically went away after they drank the potion. Their saggy breasts sprung up and looked as perky as if they were preparing to salute someone.

As these two women aged, their bodies were routinely injured and required lots of emergency repairs, which were done with a home repair kit of glue and spray. For emergencies, they carried cans of tan-colored spray paint with them in their handbags. It was really funny. Here were two ladies who definitely could have used the kind of signs that I had threatened to hang around my neck!

The message of the movie was clear to me. Vanity will kill you, or at least make you wish you were dead. Some people will do anything to try to ensure that their youth is retained for as long as possible. Growing old gracefully is not a slogan for all people, and is definitely not spoken by those who are vain.

Now that I had personally walked by death's door, my own goal had been revised. I was simply happy that I could grow old. Gracefully would be nice, but it was no longer a requirement. Longevity was the name of the game. Quality of life was my new slogan. Fate had already prevented me from having to face the irreversible effects that "Cooper's Droop" would have on my left breast if I lived to be older than fifty. The Cooper's ligaments that support my right breast might give way by then, but the left one had been spared the experience.

I had lots of visitors, including Al's family and mutual friends. Jack came by daily on his way home from work. He celebrated each step of my progress with us. Al and I talked a lot about the possible reactions that some of our friends might have. He was concerned that people would be at a loss for words and might feel uncomfortable talking about my illness.

He also worried that when people glanced at my chest it would upset me. I had all of these thoughts, too, and knew that it was perfectly natural for people to drop their eyes to my chest. It was almost an compulsive reaction, and I didn't find it offensive—I expected it. But I must admit that for those friends who didn't take a "quick peek" while I was looking at them, my respect and admiration clicked up a point or two in their favor.

The stuff-and-fluff bra turned out to really confuse some visitors, too. No one asked me which side had been removed. I'm sure that some people made bets about which side it was, and tried desperately to figure it out. Between my loosely fitting shirts and my cotton batting, it was hard to tell unless someone paid close attention and was able to notice that things I had routinely done with my left hand I now did with my right.

Our friends Jack and Linda Murphy came by to visit us one evening. This was truly one of the most enjoyable evenings during my recovery. Jack and I have been close for years, and his wife is as wonderful a person as he is. They brought me flowers and a huge beach towel with my name embroidered on it. "We want you to be getting ready for the beach as soon as you are able, so we can all spend some time in the sun on the sandy beach of Ocean City."

They didn't ask me any questions about my health, but instead waited for me to bring up the subject. We spent about two hours together talking and laughing. Though I was very tired when they left that evening, it was a lovely night that I will remember. Jack had lost his brother to cancer not long before I was diagnosed, and it was painfully clear that he didn't want to lose me, too. After they left that evening, Al and I talked about how blessed we were to have such dear friends.

Shirley stopped by quite often. She wouldn't stay very long, so as not to tire me out, and she always knew just what to say. I often cried when she came. That is one of Shirley's best features—letting friends cry on her shoulder and giving them comfort and complete acceptance. She lets you know that crying is very acceptable behavior in her presence. Being a nurse, she also knew what I had been through surgically.

Shirley is a very large-busted woman, and she was empathic about the fact that part of my image had always included my breasts. Once, when she and I were taking a walk in the woods, we suddenly realized that we had unknowingly walked through a bed of ticks. They were literally everywhere—on our pants, shirts, arms, socks, and shoes. We were furiously trying to remove as many as we could see on each other. We resorted to removing our shirts to get the ticks that had climbed into our clothing. Although we were only about twenty feet from the main road, modesty was the last thing on our minds. We continued to remove ticks and found them on our bras and even in our bras!

When we hastily returned to the cottage where we were staying, our husbands came up from the waterfront to see why we were back so soon. Privately they each assisted us in removing any remaining ticks that were on our backs, behind our ears, and in our undergarments. They found our story most entertaining and regretted they had missed our strip act on the highway. From that day forward, our husbands, Al and Jim, joked about doing "tick checks."

Obviously, it was going to be easier to check me for ticks in the future. There wouldn't be any running around lost in my cleavage anymore. My surgery had included eliminating my cleavage. Let me explain it this way—my "cleav" was gone, the "age" remained.

One evening after company had left and I was getting ready for bed, I came out of the bathroom and found Lady, our black

Labrador, lying at my feet on her big cozy bed. Lady had an unpredictable habit of running away periodically. She would jump the fence in the afternoon and not return until the wee hours of the next morning. Lady was old and had little street sense, so we would become very concerned when she didn't come home.

Lady was so old that it was a miracle she could even jump the fence. But she did, and we often spent the night worrying like the parents of a teenage girl who is out with a boy with long hair and tattoos who tells you, "Hey man, I'll get her home okay. Don't worry." The worrying begins the moment they are out of your sight, and it doesn't cease until your daughter has arrived home, is inspected for damage, and safely tucked away in bed. Only then can you turn your worry glands off.

Whenever Lady jumped the fence, the same worry glands were activated and didn't turn off until she was back inside our home lying on her bed all in one piece. I don't know exactly how much Lady understood when we talked to her, but I know she was fairly smart. She certainly knew what "dog food," "walk," "good girl," and "bad" meant.

On the evening I came out of the bathroom to find Lady lying at my feet, I was wearing just my underpants. She looked up at me, and her eyes appeared to be looking at my new incision. I bent over her and said, "Do you see this scar? Well, this is what's going to happen to you if you ever jump that fence again and run away!" The poor dog cowered down, put her tail between her legs, and crawled out to the hallway, where she slept most of the night. I felt confident I had cured her of her compulsive need to jump the fence and travel like a gypsy through the neighborhood at night.

I had made an agreement with my surgeon, Charlie Yeo, to wait until his return from vacation to get the final pathology results from my surgery. Though I would have preferred having the results sooner, Charlie preferred to review the information with me personally rather than having one of his colleagues discuss it with me in his absence. So we made a pact. I would wait for his return and would not log onto the computer myself or ask someone else at work to give me a preview of the results. Although the waiting was hard, the fear of looking at the results myself was overwhelming. I was sure that if I had logged onto the computer, the Grim Reaper's face would appear and point his ugly finger at me! It was best for me to wait.

I had an appointment with Charlie when I hit my three-week mark. It was his first day back to work, and despite his very heavy schedule, he gave me his undivided attention, as always. He also gave me the news my family and I had been waiting for: my lymph nodes were clean, and I was in stage one.

What wonderful words to hear! Everyone was thrilled with the news! It was equal to—if not more exciting than—when we announced the birth of our child twelve years before. When I think about it, we were really announcing a birth of a different nature. Perhaps it would be best to describe it as my own rebirth. I was now an official cancer survivor.

Al and I went home and called everyone to share the good news. When Al's brother, Jack, got the word, he quickly appeared at our home with a half-bushel of steamed crabs. This time there would be a happier ending for him, too. This time the person he knew so well and who shared the name Shockney, as his late wife had, would survive.

As the days passed, I felt stronger and more comfortable with my new body. At four weeks post-op, I decided it was time for Laura to have the opportunity to look at my incision. We had her sit in the middle of our bed with lots of space around her in case she fainted (which wouldn't have been any surprise to me). I slowly took off my clothes until my incision was exposed. She stared at it. She studied it and studied it, but said nothing. The silence was more than I could take so I finally asked her what she thought about it. What she said upon seeing the results of her mother's breast surgery was succinct and very powerful. She said, "I want to stay young."

I realized how hard this must have been for her to deal with. Why, it had only been a week before my surgery when I took Laura to a department store to get her fitted for bras for herself. Breasts were a major focal point in this child's mind at this particular time, and having to see her mother lose one had to be very hard. I asked her if she was worried this might happen to her and she answered, "No. Not right now I'm not worried. I might get worried when I'm older but I'm not worried right now."

I was worried though. How would I feel if I passed this kind of cancer on to my own child? Perhaps there will be a cure by the time she is my age, and she won't have to worry about this dreadful thing affecting her. I realized how important it was for her to see how I coped and adjusted to this physical loss, and how I was dealing with a diagnosis like this. If she could see that my life goes on, perhaps in an even better way than before, she might somehow benefit from the experience after all. I knew I would become active in government and local groups that were diligently working to find cures for breast cancer, as well as in providing support for those who become club members after me. Laura definitely furthered my inspiration to do what I had planned.

I received regular phone calls from Earl, my physician friend at work. He called several times a week to see how I was doing. One day I was a little down and I said, "Well, Earl, I looked in the mirror and saw what I could go as this year for Halloween. If I wear my birthday suit, I'm sure to win first prize for the scariest costume." He was another friend who knew just what to say and when to say it, so I didn't stay down in the dumps very long.

One evening when Earl called me he said he had a favor to ask. Though it had been only a few weeks since my surgery, he wondered if I would be willing to talk with a friend of his who had just that week been diagnosed with breast cancer. He thought maybe I could be of some help to her. I was flattered by his confidence in me. I also felt very excited. I was being given the opportunity to help a new club member, someone who had only been drafted into the club a few days before. My response to his request was an overwhelming "YES!"

He had her call me the following day, and she and I talked on the phone almost daily for about two weeks, which ran up to the time of her surgery. I sent her funny cards in the mail and wrote down some suggestions of things to do before as well as after her surgery. I enclosed small items in the cards that I mailed her, too, such as a packet containing a one-time application of an anti-stress facial mask, a bookmark with an inspirational phrase, a sachet for her lingerie drawer, and other feminine things that I hoped would cheer her up. They did. She was appreciative of these little gifts and cards and of my newly found words of wisdom about techniques to help her get through the days ahead. I realized that each step she took through her experience—from coping with the news of the diagnosis to her transformation surgery and getting on the road to recovery—also helped me along my own road to recovery. I realized that breast cancer survivors who were volunteers weren't only giving—they were also getting something from the women they spent time with. I knew that this new club member would be the first of many new club members I would spend time with and help along this very scary path as best I could. It was a special privilege to be asked to help and guide her, and I knew that helping others in the future would be a privilege as well.

Chapter 15

For several weeks Al spent his nights in a sleeping bag next to our bed before he felt comfortable lying in bed with me. I was worried that he would bump my chest, and he was worried about it, too. But I needed him close to me, so we resorted to his sleeping on the floor. He must have felt like he was at summer camp or something. After about two and a half weeks or so, he tested out his designated spot in the bed. I think the first night he slept beside me again, neither one of us slept very well—we were both too afraid something would go wrong. Al was already experienced in having to be careful with me in bed. I have broken many bones in our fifteen years of marriage, and he has slept beside me when I had casts on my legs and my arms, slings and immobilizers on my torso, and a variety of other contraptions that are not very conducive to sleep. We were anxious to resume our normal sleeping routine, however, so we decided to give it a try. If ever there was a time I wanted the man I loved close to me, it was now. I needed reassurance that I was loved and that the absence of my left breast wouldn't result in my being loved less.

We also talked about the best time to resume our sexual relationship. I realized it was probably best to just let nature take its course, but I had the distinct feeling I was going to derail nature's course unless things were carefully planned out. I wanted time to prepare myself. To think positive thoughts. To feel the timing was right. It was almost like starting over for me. I looked at my husband as if he were a stranger of sorts, and I felt a little unknown to him.

We planned to have an intimate encounter about three weeks after my surgery, on a night Laura planned to sleep over at a friend's house. It was very late and I was extremely nervous. Al was equally nervous. We probably looked like two teenagers fumbling in the back seat of a car. I was afraid of rejection; he was afraid of hurting me. He made every effort to be cautious, not leaning on my chest at all. I made every effort to focus on his face to see any signals that might imply that my missing breast was a turn-off.

It was a tense night. I can't say it was extremely pleasurable. It was okay. It would have been fine if I had been more trusting of Al when he told me that my mastectomy didn't make any difference to him—that it didn't make me seem like less of a woman to him. I needed proof, however, and felt this night would be the real test.

As I look back on it now, I think it was a miracle that Al was able to perform at all. If he looked the wrong way, or moved in a different manner, I questioned it. The first time was definitely the roughest, physically and emotionally. As time went by, we relied on nature taking its course again, and we were able to experience the kind of closeness and intimacy we'd had before. Al would say to me, "When I press my chest up against yours now, our hearts can be closer to one another." What a romantic thing to say.

I often thought about other club members and wondered if they had experienced the same kind of anxiety in resuming intimacy that my husband and I had experienced. I thought about the patient I had taken care of who'd had her mastectomy many years before I saw her as a patient for another medical problem. She was the patient who'd had phantom limb sensation, which I did now.

As time went by and my incision became less tender, Al would gently touch it. Before too long we were playing a new game called "In Search of the Missing Nipple." It was a fun game, and a great tension breaker on the nights that I was feeling slightly self-conscious about my new appearance.

Laura was getting adjusted to my new body, too. She would come into the bathroom while I was taking a bubble bath and look at my incision. She even told me she had gotten used to seeing me with only one breast, and thought I looked pretty good that way. (Kids are amazing, aren't they? So resilient. So honest. Always pressing forward.)

When I hit six weeks, I was eligible to be fitted for a breast prosthesis. Good-bye stuff-and-fluff! I had made an appointment at the store called We Fit, only about twenty minutes from my home. They recommend taking someone along when you are fitted, someone you are close to who will give you an honest critique of how the prosthesis looks on you. You don't want someone who is the type to always say, "Oh, that looks fine," when everyone else thinks it looks silly. You know, Dolly Parton on one side and Peter Pan on the other. I decided to take my mother.

Al was disappointed that I had not decided to take him, but I told him I felt it was important to take a woman with me. I'd be in a room with other mastectomy patients, and the store recommended that I bring a woman I could trust to give me useful and accurate feedback about how I looked in the various prostheses that I would try on. If you can't trust your mother, who can you trust?

Besides, I felt this would be a positive experience for her, too. She was still so worried about me. Wishing that none of this had happened to me. Wanting to make it all go away. Somehow wanting to be able to make me whole again. When I called and asked her if she would be willing to go with me, she said she would be honored to.

Mom and I arrived at We Fit at about 10:00 a.m. The shop was very busy that morning with lots of women buying all kinds of undergarments. This particular store sells all sorts of lingerie, underpants, bras, girdles, etc., and they specialize in women who are hard to fit. One of the items someone was picking up for a bridal shower was a black lace teddy in size 4X —not the size you usually associate with these kinds of garments. I approached the counter and told the lady behind the desk I was there for a prosthesis fitting. She ushered me to the back of the store where the fitting rooms were located. Mom followed.

When I got into the dressing area, the woman waiting on us introduced herself as Miriam. An older woman, she was very soft-spoken. She asked how long it had been since my surgery so she could confirm that I was at least six weeks post-op. She also asked if my surgeon had okayed my fitting, and I handed her my prescription from his office. (The prescription simply said to fit me for a breast prosthesis. It didn't limit the particular kind or anything else. Surgeons are smart enough to leave those choices to the fitter and the patient.)

Miriam asked me to undress from the waist up, which I did. She stood looking at me with no surprise at all as I exposed my ten-inch incision, which stretched across my chest from my breastbone to my armpit. She stared at my incision for a second or two, then said, "You look like a forty-two C or D. I think you'll take an Amoena, size nine."

Size nine? What was she talking about? Was I buying Italian shoes or an artificial breast? She stepped over to a huge closet and opened its French doors. Inside were hundreds of boxes that looked like oversized shoeboxes. I read the writing on their sides. "Amoena size 9 left." "Amoena size 7 right." There were literally hundreds of prosthesis in this closet! All shapes and sizes, and a variety of brands.

Miriam took down three boxes, a size eight, nine, and ten, and brought them to my dressing room. She had me try on a mastectomy bra as well. She put the size nine prosthesis in the pocket of the bra and gave it to me to try on. It felt clumsy at first, because the bra was so heavy on one side from the weight of the prosthesis. I put it on and Miriam checked the fit. I was instructed to put on the fitted knit shirt I had brought with me to see how the new breast looked compared to its real mate. It was important that the contour of my figure look symmetrical and that the size of the prosthesis match the size of my natural breast.

I looked into the mirror intently. This was a very important purchase for me, and it required undivided attention. I also tried on the size eight and the size ten. Mom gave her opinion about how each one looked to her. She was very intent, as I was, and wanted the fit to be absolutely perfect. Miriam was right when she had originally looked me over and sized me up. Size nine was the best fit. I tried it on again, this time with more confidence and a feeling of peace of mind.

Mom looked at me just as she had when I was fitted for my

wedding gown. She wanted everything to be perfect. She wanted me to feel beautiful. And I did. Mom said, "You look whole again. I can sleep tonight." It was a good day for both of us.

I had a real appreciation for the skills Miriam possessed. Being able to merely glance at my chest and know instinctively what size and shape of breast prosthesis I would best look in seemed to me truly amazing. Now I better understand why they call these people "fitters." I also had an appreciation for the club members who had come before me, because they had given Miriam the ability to easily complete this task and sort through the volume of oversized shoe boxes in that closet. The Boob Closet.

Miriam cautioned me to wear my prosthesis regularly. She said some women buy them and then put them away in the box and don't wear them. I found this surprising. Since that time, however, I've met a lot of other mastectomy patients who have experienced trouble with their own prosthesis, which has resulted in their switching to other brands or going without. Small-breasted women can have trouble with the prosthesis floating around in the pocket of their bras. Large-breasted women like myself are sometimes troubled with the weight of the prosthesis.

Because the prostheses are made out of silicone and are solid matter, they don't give your skin an opportunity to breathe and can cause excessive sweating. I've had trouble with this myself, and am busy with patenting what I hope will be a remedy for all mastectomy patients who suffer with the same problem. I definitely didn't want to have this very special item sitting in a box at home. I considered my prosthesis just as important as some people feel their American Express card is—I don't leave home without it!

Mom and I headed home to show Al how I looked. He was beaming when he saw me. He said, "Now which one has the Toni?"

I pointed to the right side and said, "This one is the live one; the left side is the Memorex version."

Al could see I had my confidence back. I stood taller now and walked without worrying that someone could tell I'd had a breast removed. I laughed to myself that night in bed about my pre-operative trips to the shopping centers, searching for fake boobs on other women. There was no doubt in my mind that I had probably seen quite a few boobs that were prosthetic versions of the real thing. These women had been to see Miriam or some other fitter at a mastectomy supply shop that carried breast forms.

Prostheses no longer look like jellyfish, as they used to twenty-five years ago. They look quite natural, and when inside a bra can pass for the real thing without any trouble. There were times that Al still forgot about my surgery or which side it was on and grabbed my left side for a quick and risqué squeeze, only to find that I didn't respond to his touch because he'd gotten the wrong side! I showed Jack my prosthesis. He was very impressed, and asked me if he could sleep with her sometime.

You may have noticed that I refer to the prosthesis as her. That's because I decided to name my prosthesis. I chose a name even before I chose her. Her name is Betty. Betty Boob, to be precise. I figured that choosing a prosthesis was similar to choosing a puppy. She was going to become a family member and would be spending a lot of time with me. Everywhere that I went, Betty was sure to go. She deserved a name of her own. After all, she was my bosom buddy, right?

My friend Wanda from Virginia brought me a special present when she came to visit shortly after I had gotten Betty. It was a ceramic Christmas ornament that she had specially made for me. It was shaped like a baby bottle and had inscribed on it, "Betty Boob's first Christmas, 1992." Christmas was several months away, but I chose not to wait for our tree to be put up before I displayed this precious welcoming gift. I hung it in our entryway, and it became quite a conversation piece. I still enjoy it!

About two weeks after I got Betty I went back to We Fit and was fitted for a mastectomy bathing suit and a swimmer's breast prosthesis. Swimmer's prostheses are lighter in weight and made of a special foam that contains buckshot in the center to provide a little bit of weight.

I heard that when the company first came out with the swimmer's model, it was made out of Styrofoam and didn't function well. Apparently when a woman got in the water, the prosthesis served as a flotation device. Perhaps the device would have been useful if the woman was learning how to swim or had fallen overboard, but for everyday use in a swimming pool it was a loser. The next version released was made of foam rubber. It was equally awful because it absorbed water like a sponge. Not only would it pull a woman down in the water, but when she attempted to get out of the pool, her "breast" would be hanging at about waist level and spurting water. I can see these poor women saying, "Please excuse me while I go wring out my breast."

I was definitely fortunate that the trials and testing of a swimming model were over. I was able to leave We Fit with a swimmer's model size two. It works quite well—or should I say that she works quite well? Yes, she has a name, too. Surely you can guess the name of Betty's swimming partner. For those of you who can't, her name is Esther. Esther Williams. Who did you expect?

Since adding Betty and Esther to our family tree, I have had the opportunity to get information about some other prostheses on the market. A friend of mine about my age who had a mastectomy several years ago sent me some literature and a videotape about a fairly new design of prosthesis. It's becoming increasingly popular with women who have had a mastectomy and are average- to small-breasted.

The breast prosthesis sticks onto a woman's chest wall with Velcro. Yes, that's right. Velcro. A very creative person figured out how to use the same kind of adhesive that is used for attaching ostomy bags to a patient's skin and decided to try it out on women who don't want to worry about a prosthesis contained in a pocket.

The woman applies a special adhesive tape that is non-irritating to the skin. The exterior side of the tape has Velcro on it. The inner portion of the breast prosthesis also has Velcro on it, which adheres to the Velcro strip on the tape. The company that makes this prosthesis is called Colorplast. The woman just presses the prosthesis in place and voilà! She has a prosthesis that doesn't require a bra to keep it in place!

From feedback I've received from other women this is a great model, but not very practical for large-breasted women. The Velcro works to a point, but the weight of the prosthesis for a woman of my bust size causes the skin to pull at the adhesive application site. That's okay, because Betty and I are doing just fine anyway.

Al and I thought that if ever I changed my mind and I decided to get this stick-on model, he would help me stick it on. Of course, we weren't thinking about applying it using the techniques shown in the videotape. Instead, we thought it would be great fun to have Al stand back from me about ten feet, and, using the techniques of a baseball pitcher, throw it into place. Perhaps we could even keep score! Four. Strike one! Well, as I've said before, humor has gotten us through many a bad day and night, and this is just another example of it.

I gave Al a request for Christmas. I told him that this company also sold stick-on nipples. You could buy them in various skin tone shades, as well as different diameter measurements. I told him that if he needed any gift ideas for the holidays, stick-on nipples sure would make a unique stocking stuffer!

Chapter 16

Returning to work was exciting, but I became fatigued easily. I expected my body to work at my usual pace of sixty hours a week, and it refused to cooperate.

It was marvelous to see everyone. My staff and coworkers were very glad to see me back and relieved I was doing well. I think working with so many women added a great deal to my support system. Don't get me wrong, the men I work with and am very close to were certainly there for me, too, when the chips were down. It's just that the women I am close to and see every day could relate better to what I was going through. Of course, each one of them, I'm sure, was hoping she would not be the next in the one-out-of-eight statistic to have the same experience.

It felt wonderful to get so many hugs. I didn't feel completely confident hugging people, but now my stuff-and-fluff cotton batting prosthesis had been replaced by my permanent one, Betty.

I sent a lot of letters to family and friends during my six-week recovery period. I not only wrote thank-you notes for the thoughtful flowers, cards, and gifts that people sent me, I also wrote special sentimental letters, thanking each one for her or his support during my tough times. I wanted to let people know I was a fighter and had no plans of giving up and letting the Big C get me. Holding onto optimism was key, and sharing those thoughts was an uplifting experience for me.

Under other circumstances I might not have sent such letters—I would have considered it too corny or something. But it felt very natural and oh so right to do that now.

I wanted people to know that I appreciated them, that their thoughtfulness and caring were a big part of my ability to recover so well. With their love, I had hope. With their friendship, I had a future. This had been an experience. I was dealt a hand that showed me what I would get when I didn't get what I wanted. But it also was a learning experience for me. I learned that life is precious, that my marriage could survive an awful blow, and that with God's love and the support of friends and family, I'd get through this crisis.

I frequently reflect on the good fortune of being spared chemotherapy because of my lymph nodes testing negative. While I was getting well, our long-time friend John Cross was getting sicker. He had a craniotomy done in an attempt to remove a malignant brain tumor. The operation proved only partially successful.

While I gradually improved, John's health gradually declined. He and his wife, Pat, visited us frequently. We saw them a lot once he agreed to have his medical care transferred from the small-town hospital where they lived to Johns Hopkins Hospital. We were able to provide him with the very best surgical and medical oncology treatment that could be offered, but his gliosarcoma was a grade IV and would not respond to treatment. I visited his room daily. He and I had bonded like siblings. He always wanted to know how I was doing, what my blood work results showed, how my X-rays looked. He told me that he wanted me to be "one hundred percent."

"If I have to lose some so that you can gain some, that's all right with me. I want you to be well again and stay well."

I watched this man slowly slip away. I watched his wife of more than twenty-five years become emotionally shattered and the rest of his family suffer. He died in the small town where he had lived nearly all his life. I elected not to attend his funeral, even though my husband was a pallbearer. I feared that seeing him lying in a casket would be more than I could take. We had both battled cancer together. I was afforded the opportunity to be a survivor; he was not. This was not due to his lack of will power or desire, but solely to the progression of the disease and God's will. I miss John to this day, but feel that somehow he is looking down on me, doing whatever is in his power so he can be my guardian angel.

By November 1992, I was three and a half months into my recovery. Things were progressing along as scheduled until one morning when I was in the shower. I felt a lump in my other breast.

Oh no, I thought. This can't be happening to me. Why is this happening to me?

The timing was awful—not that there is ever a good time to find a lump in one's breast. On this particular morning the hospital was due for an inspection by the Joint Commission. This is an accrediting body that grants the hospital approval for providing care to Medicare, Medicaid, and Blue Cross recipients. The commission evaluates and scores the quality of care provided to our patients based on the records we keep. The function of record-keeping rests primarily with my office. This organization comes once every three years, and today was the first day of a five-day inspection.

When I got to work, I called to make an appointment with Charlie. I was due for a mammogram at the end of the week, so I decided to leave the X-ray schedule as it was rather than change it to an earlier time. I wanted to get through the accreditation inspection first, then deal with my own personal problems. If the lump was cancerous, it had just appeared. If it was something benign, it could wait. I decided to use this external agency inspection as a diversion from my medical problems.

The inspection went well. As a matter of fact, the areas I was responsible for, including medical staff quality assessment and utilization management, received very high scores. As soon as the folks were out the door, I was in the hands of the radiology folks again so I could find out what this lump was. All I could think about was that Betty was about to have a roommate. I'd have two oversized shoe boxes with breast prostheses in them. I guess I'd be calling them the Boobsy Twins.

A mammogram was done. I was very nervous during the procedure. Once again, I asked if my radiologist friend was available to be with me. He arrived shortly after I made the request. Al was waiting in the reception area for me. He had hives on his face, as usual. The female radiologist entered the room and said, "It looks like a cyst. I suggest that we make sure by doing an ultrasound exam. If it is a cyst, then it should probably be drained." A cyst. Well, that sounded good to me. Take me to ultrasound and let's get on with this business!

In the ultrasound room, the machine that is used is much kinder than the jaws of the mammography machine. The mass visualized on the screen did contain liquid. The next step was to drain the cyst. When Charlie had originally drained the cyst (which was the same one—it had refilled and gotten a little bit larger this time), he had simply stuck a tiny needle in it and poof, it was gone. But for some reason, this time the procedure wasn't so simple.

My breast was placed back in the mammography machine, and this time converted into a waffle. The radiologist then inserted the needle, and the pressure of the machine squeezing my breast caused the needle to automatically fill with fluid from the cyst. It was painful. I kept thinking that when the radiologist pulled the needle out, my breast would still be spouting fluid like an erupting volcano. It didn't, though. By taking before-and-after pictures on the ultrasound machine, she confirmed that the cyst was completely empty. I left the radiology suite with a sore chest and a big smile.

Al was greatly relieved. Our radiologist friend had already been talking with him while I was having the aspiration done. Just another dress rehearsal, I guess, but one that haunted me. Was it just a rehearsal for the real thing again? You know, like the movie *Poltergeist*. What did the little girl say in that film? "They're baaaaaaack."

I saw Charlie a few days later. He reviewed my radiology pictures and seemed satisfied that the lump was a cyst, but he added a little caution to his remarks. He told me that although the pathology report showed cystic fluid, there was no guarantee that cancer cells weren't present. He recommended that if the cyst refilled once more, I have a lumpectomy. He told me I would be on his list of close surveillance patients in the future.

I told him how much the fear of recurrence worried me. He appreciated my concern and discussed the option of having a prophylactic mastectomy done. This would be my choice, of course. If I started dreading each day because I worried about a recurrence, it might be a smart thing to do. I decided to hold this option in reserve for now. Why have surgery if you don't absolutely have to?

Since that visit in November, I have met several women who have chosen preventive measures to keep them from worrying every day about the possibility of recurrence. Each seemed pleased with her choice. For now, I thought, I'll take the breast self-exam route and try to think more optimistically.

It certainly made me envious of that medical device the doctor used on the old *Star Trek* reruns. Bones, as I believe he was nick-named, would hold a little machine that looked like a small calculator over an ill person, and within a few seconds the machine would chirp. Then he'd say, "It appears that this man is infected with a potentially deadly virus that is carried by a small insect found only on the planet Wolitble. I'll give him an injection of Smoglot. He'll be fine in a moment or two." Wouldn't it be won-derful to own such a device? They'd be selling them at K-Mart as a blue-light special.

I didn't see my friend Lynda until Christmas week to show her how Betty and I looked as a team. We were at Charles and Lynda's home for dinner, and she and I went into their bedroom for a show-and-tell session. I showed her my incision first. She looked intrigued and was impressed with the narrowness of my scar. I truly do have excellent skin, which promotes good healing. A gene my father blessed me with. My mother's surgical scars are very wide; her body unfortunately makes keloids.

Lynda held my prosthesis. She said, "Why, it feels just like a breast! This is amazing! See, I told you that you would do fine. This is merely an inconvenience, but it's not you. It's just flesh. Our Lillie is still here. Thank God!"

Laura became more inquisitive about my prosthesis, too. One evening I found her in the bathroom holding it up to her chest, eval-uating her appearance in the mirror. I said, "Laura, what are you doing with my breast prosthesis?" She glanced up at me, com-pletely startled at my entering the bathroom and finding her in this odd situation. She said, "I was just wondering. If my breasts don't get as big as I want them to be, can any woman buy these, or can you only get them if you've had a breast removed for cancer? I think this thing is pretty neat. The boys would love it. Just look at how big I'd look if I wore yours!" I just shook my head and laughed. I assured her that her breasts would probably grow to a size that met her expectations and to not worry about it. But to answer her question I told her yes, any woman can buy these.

From the time I had been diagnosed up until about six months after my surgery, I had a lot of people ask me whether or not I planned to have reconstructive surgery. I felt very uncomfortable with this chronic question. I wasn't bothered by the asking as much as by the way in which some people chose to make the inquiry. "Are you planning to have reconstruction? I had a friend who did and she is really happy with the results." Or, "I know someone who had to have it undone, poor thing. You aren't looking to have it done, are you?" These questions didn't bother me.

But one did: "You are going to have reconstruction, aren't you?" This was said in a way that implied something was wrong with me if I didn't have it done. On numerous occasions, I was tempted to respond in a less-than-friendly manner. Rather than giving my usual reply, "Al and I have discussed it and I've opted not to have it done at this time, and probably never will," perhaps I could have said instead, "No, I'm not. I've heard that you've had your face lifted and your nose fixed and obviously you didn't get your money's worth, so I'm steering clear of plastic surgery for now."

I did give a lot of thought to reconstruction, though. It seems that so many women have chosen it. I was not a candidate for implants, but was and still am a candidate for a tram flap procedure. This procedure involves having your abdominal tissue and blood vessels removed from your belly and placed in your chest. The result is a breast mound that simulates a real breast. If the woman waits several months before having reconstruction, she has had some time to adjust to the loss and is more content with its simulated replacement.

I based my own decision on a multitude of things. First, I didn't want to undergo surgery that wasn't necessary and carried risk. Second, I wanted to know how important a facsimile version of a breast would be to my husband. He made it clear that it made no difference to him. Third, I asked Laura about her opinion. She was quite clear on her feelings about reconstructive surgery.

She said, "No. I don't think you should have it done. Nothing can replace your breast. It's gone. Moving your tummy tissue up to your chest doesn't give you a new breast. It just covers up your scar by relocating skin and tissue that belongs someplace else. You look fine as you are. You should stay this way. Betty looks fine on you."

So my decision was made. I may change my mind some time in the future, but I doubt it. I also feared that some day the other shoe would drop and I'd have to have another mastectomy done. If this were to occur, I wouldn't have achieved anything by having my left breast rebuilt. There would be nothing left to provide a reconstruction of the right side. So I decided to be content with Betty, and continued to take advantage of the phantom limb sensation I have. The sensation would be lost if I had reconstruction. No more playing our game of "In Search of the Missing Nipple." Well then, forget it!

I do respect the wishes and desires of other club members who choose to utilize this option of reconstruction. It's marvelous that women nowadays have a choice. Knowing that I have a choice and can exercise it in the future, if I so desire, is a good feeling.

Since my mastectomy was done in 1992, dramatic improvements have been made in breast reconstructive surgery. A procedure called "skin sparing mastectomy with tram flap reconstruction" is now being done, and the results are amazing. The breast is hollowed out and the nipple removed, keeping the outer skin of the breast intact. The abdominal fat (that's the tram flap part of the procedure) is used to refill the breast. After nipple tattooing is completed and a few months pass post-op, you can hardly tell that any surgery occurred. And more research is now underway to develop methods to give sensation to this new breast. Although that isn't possible yet, in time, we believe, it will be. Amazing!

Chapter 17

Traveling with a prosthesis is an adventure unto itself. The first few trips away from home are an experience and worth mentioning. I had my first opportunity to travel with Betty on an overnight business trip during Thanksgiving week. I went to Philadelphia for a consulting assignment at a large teaching hospital. It was my first experience carrying heavy objects (my briefcase and suitcase). I realized that my arm was not as strong as I thought it was. I felt doubly disadvantaged because my good arm wasn't so good anymore because I'd broken my right shoulder the year before my mastectomy surgery. I somehow muddled through with the assistance of Advil.

When I got to my hotel room, I discovered that instead of a king-sized bed as I had anticipated, the room had two double beds. Normally I would have called down to the front desk and requested to be relocated to another room, but this time I decided I wouldn't bother. Who knows, maybe Betty had changed the reservations, since she knew she was going on her first out-of-town adventure. When I got ready for bed that night, I didn't put Betty in the box she was usually stored in at home. Boxes are not conducive to travel; a box for a breast prosthesis would have required its own suitcase just for traveling!

I decided that just for the fun of it, I'd put Betty in the other double bed all by herself. If I had had access to a pair of stick-on eyes and a plastic fake nose, I would have put them on her and taken her picture. As it was, I was laughing myself to sleep anyway, think of how silly I was to put my prosthesis in her own bed. But it was fun. I was in the privacy of my own hotel room, and the only way anyone would know that I had done such a silly thing would be if the fire alarm required a rapid evacuation of the building.

Even under such circumstances, I think I would probably have grabbed my pocketbook and Betty before leaving my room. Since there was no such emergency that night, Betty and I each rested well, she in her own bed with pretty sheets, a blanket, and a gorgeous bedspread, and I in mine.

My next adventure with Betty was when we went to Disney World in April 1993. For this trip I also took my swimmer's breast prosthesis, Esther. I had purchased a new mastectomy bathing suit and was eager to try out my new prosthesis.

We spent our third day at Typhoon Lagoon, a water park contained within Disney World. It has slides, swimming holes, a wave machine, and (my favorite) a relaxing ride that takes you in an inner tube floating downstream for about a quarter of a mile. The ride is in Castaway Creek, and takes you in a giant circle around the park. I loved it. Esther seemed content, too. I rode around in the inner tube for about an hour, then got out to get some lunch.

It's funny how self-conscious you feel when you're wearing something new, particularly if the new item is a breast. By the time I had gotten something to eat, walked around the park to watch the kids screaming their heads off in the wave rider machine, and walked back to our staked-out area where we had left our towels and bags, I felt everyone at the water park had looked at my chest. I knew it was all in my mind and I was simply being overly self-conscious about my new bathing suit and prosthesis, but nonetheless I felt as if people were staring at my chest with a look of puzzlement. It wasn't until later in the day when I went to the bathroom that I realized my paranoia had a valid explanation behind it.

I got to the bathroom and waited in line for an empty stall. While waiting, I glanced in the mirror to see how I looked in my new bathing suit and to see how much sun I had gotten on my back. Good heavens! Esther had moved! That's right, moved. I don't mean to imply she wasn't there anymore (she hadn't moved out), but she had gotten herself twisted up somehow and was definitely not where she belonged. Rather than being a symmetrical match to my real breast, Esther had dropped lower and turned herself from a horizontal position to a vertical one! No wonder people were looking at me!

Needless to say, during my turn in the stall I rearranged Esther back into position. I decided there was no reason to get upset about it. I actually found it kind of funny, and I learned the importance of making sure that a swimmer's prosthesis doesn't have a lot of room to move about. That's what the problem was. When I was in the inner tube, my arms were in an odd position, so the prosthesis had shuffled itself around and changed its position, thereby changing its shape.

When we got back to our hotel room, I sewed the pocket of the mastectomy bra smaller to prevent Esther's moving around and changing her position in the future. What a funny day!

During the same week that we went to Disney World, I decided to write a special letter to someone. That special person was Erma Bombeck. I had read her article in *Redbook* magazine about her experience with breast cancer and had seen portions of her article again in *Reader's Digest*. I was really pleased that someone as professionally visible and famous as she was would let the world know she had become a club member several years before.

I wrote how much I admired her for coming forth and telling the world about her mastectomy surgery. I also told her I hoped that as a result of her having done so, other women would be inspired to get a mammogram and do breast self-exams as well. I also shared some of the funny experiences that had occurred to me during the period from my diagnosis to treatment and thereafter.

I sent my letter inside an Easter card. I felt this particular card was perfect for me to send to her. As a matter of fact, I bought two more of the same card and sent one to my surgeon, Charlie Yeo, and one to my secretary, Diane. The front of the card depicted an elderly woman with a large bosom holding a basket full of Easter eggs. The message said, "This year I'm going to hide the Easter eggs where no one will ever think to look." Inside the card it said, "In my bra."

Three weeks after I sent Erma my letter, she wrote back. I was flattered that she would take the time to respond, and I felt that much closer to someone else who had traveled the scary path required to become a breast cancer survivor. She confirmed for me the value of humor as a real healer, and how important it is not to be silent about the disease.

The more people who know there are lots of club members out there, the quicker we will encourage more women to take advantage of preventive medical care. I hope the knowledge will also promote awareness within the government and medical research organizations so that adequate research money is allocated to the treatment and prevention of breast cancer. It would be wonderful if we could find a cure to rid ourselves of this disease once and for all.

By the time we returned from our Disney World vacation, it had been almost a year since my original biopsy had started me down the path of transformation. I could hardly believe it had been almost a year. This meant I would soon be due for my annual gynecological exam, as well as my first official annual mammogram and visit to my surgeon.

First came the gyn exam. No sweat. I wasn't at all concerned. I felt fine. I had no new menstrual problems. The exam should be a snap. No problem. Right? Wrong. While my gynecologist was examining me, he noted that my right ovary was slightly enlarged and very tender. I'd also had blood work done the week before, and the results showed an elevated testosterone level. Oh-oh. Not what I expected.

He said, "I think in view of your history of breast cancer it would be wise to have some additional tests done to make sure that what we're seeing right now isn't ovarian cancer. I know this is not what you want to hear, but I think we need to exercise some caution here. I'll get you scheduled for a transvesical/transvaginal ultrasound procedure so we can visualize the ovaries and see what the problem is."

Definitely not what I had planned to hear. When a man has his head in your crotch, the only thing that a woman wants to hear are positive things about herself, not comments that sound negative. Oh well. I realized I was about to undergo another experience.

Chapter 18

When I got home that evening, I told Al my news. He said he felt nauseated and had to leave the dinner table for a moment. I prayed to God that whatever this problem was, please don't let it be ovarian cancer. Ovarian cancer makes breast cancer look like a simple case of acne. It is deadly. The survival rate is poor. I didn't want to think I had just weathered the storm of breast cancer only to be swept away by its wicked stepsister, ovarian cancer.

My ultrasound procedure was two weeks later. For those of you who haven't had the opportunity to experience such a procedure, it is somewhere in the family with mammography. A large "wand" that looks like a dildo in disguise is inserted into the vaginal canal until it touches your tonsils. Now that might seem pleasurable to some, but not to me, especially since it is required that the patient have a full bladder. A very full bladder. However, I was able to get the results right away.

Hooray! It was an ovarian cyst! When I got the news that it was an ovarian cyst I felt like performing a college football cheer by doing cartwheels in the hall, shouting, "Give me a C, give me a Y, give me an S, give me a T!"

Compared with hearing the word "cancer" being uttered from the radiologist's mouth, learning I had only a cyst made me absolutely thrilled! The cyst was small and the radiologist said it should be no problem. There was no explanation as to why my testosterone was so high, however. Testosterone, of course, is a male hormone. Both sexes carry some levels of both male and female hormones in their bodies. My testosterone was higher than the norm.

I concluded that it was because of the environment I worked in. When you are in the center of a political arena and the players you are contending with are mostly male, it is probably useful to have

an elevated testosterone level. I've read that some women with elevated testosterone levels got them as a result of having to compete
with men in high executive positions. Perhaps that is what had happened to me. I spend my work day in a highly politically charged
environment surrounded by doctors, the majority of whom are
men. Maybe my body was secretly growing its own three-piece set
to keep up with the big boys. I really didn't care. I was just relieved
I didn't have cancer again. So were my family and friends.

A few weeks later while I was in the shower, I felt something
else in my right breast: a knot. Coincidentally, it was in the same
location where—at the same time the previous year—I had developed the breast pain that caused me to get the first mammogram.
The knot felt like an almond and was very hard. I was due for my
annual mammogram in five weeks, so I decided to watch it until
then and not to panic about it. It was probably just another cyst. No
big deal. It remained there consistently, even during my periods,
and by the time of my mammogram, it was slightly larger in size.

I had the mammogram on the morning of June 23. Al drove from
home to be with me for the procedure. He patiently stayed in the
waiting room while I had pictures taken. The radiologist felt the
lump but was unable to visualize it on the films. She said, "Your
breast tissue is very dense," which I had heard before as an explanation of why the mass wasn't showing up on the films. I'm not
sure if it's a compliment or a criticism, but I've always taken it as
a compliment of sorts because women who are young are usually
the ones with dense breast tissue.

Since the mammogram was inconclusive, I was taken to ultrasound to see if the lump could be visualized there. I thought that it
would, because I thought it was a cyst. Wishful thinking on my
part. But no cyst visualized. The radiologist told me she would
have another doctor look at the films, but they would probably be
recommending a biopsy to be sure it wasn't another primary tumor.

My heart sank. When I got dressed and went to the waiting
room, Al could see I was not a happy camper. I told him the news.
He kissed me and told me that no matter what the outcome, we'd

be all right.

I asked him to call my folks with the news. I was sticking to my bargain, which was to keep them informed, even though I really didn't want to give them any more bad news. I could already picture my mother's face when she heard Al's report, complete with droopy left eyelid due to the sudden development of a severe migraine headache. That's why I thought it was best for him to talk with them. Somehow he has a calming effect on people. He can give you news that really isn't too good to hear and not make it sound like the end of the world.

I remember when he called me at work three years ago and very calmly told me that he and Laura had just survived a major tornado at our home. I wasn't even upset to hear him tell me, and didn't realize the full impact of the situation until I got home and discovered other people's roofs and kitchen curtains in our backyard! The place looked like we had just been bombed by a military enemy! But Al was perfectly calm. It's good to have someone like that during crisis moments, isn't it?

I already had an appointment with Charlie Yeo on July 1. I didn't feel the need to try to move it ahead. It was less than a week away, which would give the radiology department time to have my films reread by another doctor. It would also give me time to collect myself and think about the possible consequences of the next step.

This was not what I had pictured happening on my first anniversary as a breast cancer survivor. Just when I thought it was over, or at least when I'd hoped it was over, it wasn't. If this was merely another dress rehearsal, how many more dress rehearsals would there be in my future? Would there never be true closure to my experience with breast cancer?

I realized I already knew the answer, but it had been carefully and strategically pushed far to the back of my brain. No, there would never be complete closure. Once breast cancer touches you, you are always watchful for its return.

I think this is one of the reasons why women often wait a year or even longer before they start attending breast cancer support meetings. They have the support they need while going through the actual crisis of receiving the diagnosis and going through the surgery, even chemo and radiation. But once a year of time has passed and the immediate crisis is over, some part of a woman's brain chronically fears the return of the disease or the visitation of one of its relatives, like ovarian cancer, lung cancer, or bone cancer. I've seen it on the faces of women I've talked with who are members of support groups.

On this particular night, I saw a very clear picture of what a woman looked like who was afraid that cancer had returned. She was staring back at me from the bathroom mirror.

Once again, my family and coworkers were there to support me. Marge, one of my staff who also happens to be the wife of a minister, was especially supportive during the time between my mammogram and my actually getting to see my surgeon. Bryanna, another of my staff, who is like a sister to me, had the opportunity to see Charlie during that week and, with my permission, gave him a capsule version of what was going on with me. He was prepared to see a Nervous Nellie in the exam room on July 1.

My secretary, Diane, was in a state of denial about the whole thing. I didn't talk much about it because I was afraid she would cry, and if she cried I knew that I would soon be standing in a bucket of tears right beside her. Scott was also very supportive. Everyone wanted all of this awfulness that seemed to keep happening to me to go away.

I saw Charlie during my lunch break. I had picked up my mammography and ultrasound films from radiology so he could see them. He already had a printed copy of what the radiologist's reading of the films had shown. He spent a lot of time examining me, focusing intently on the hard lump that had appeared only six weeks before. His advice was the same as that of the radiology physicians. A biopsy was the only way for us to know for sure what it really was. He said he would schedule me for an open excisional biopsy under local anesthesia, with some IV sedation, in about ten days.

I called Al and told him the plans for outpatient surgery. The procedure was scheduled during our vacation week. I'm sure if I had told Charlie I was to be on vacation during that week, he would have booked me for later in the month, but I didn't want to wait. I wanted to get it over with so I knew what I was dealing with.

Laura was distressed when I told her I had to have another biopsy. She said, "Tell them that you've had enough done. I don't want you losing the other breast. One is enough." She was without humor that evening. She looked serious and acted serious. I caught her staring at me frequently while we sat together in the living room watching a movie on television. I don't know what she was thinking. Quite frankly, I was afraid to ask.

Al and I talked a lot during that Fourth of July weekend. The previous year at that time he was consoling me about the mastectomy surgery I was scheduled to have when we returned from vacationing in Maine. Now he was consoling me about the possibility of having biopsy results that might send me down a path resulting in a new roommate for Betty. He knew I didn't want to lose my other breast.

I was trying to brace myself for the results, no matter what the outcome. I explained to Al that Charlie might end up doing a lumpectomy during the biopsy. If the biopsy was positive and my breast became smaller, I might need to get a prosthesis a size or two smaller than Betty. She was a size nine, and was definitely a pretty hefty girl. Though she came with a two-year warranty, she didn't come with a trade-in policy. I doubted she would be a very popular item at a yard sale. Or perhaps she would draw a good crowd to a yard sale—you know, like tires do. Maybe I could run an ad in the newspaper to sell her. It could say:

"For sale to a good and loving home. One left-sided externally worn silicone breast prosthesis. Her name is Betty. Excellent condition. Only nine months old. Seeking a woman in need of a left breast. Still under her two-year warranty. Also still a virgin. Please call present owner for an agreeable time to see her and make offer

if interested. References required."

Well, I guess that could be an option, depending on the outcome of my biopsy. I figured there were three possibilities:

1) The procedure would be an excisional biopsy with little tissue removed. The results would be negative. No further surgery needed.

2) The procedure would involve a portion of the breast being removed, which would result in Betty being larger than her flesh-and-blood mate. If so, Betty might have to be put away in my hope chest as a souvenir of the past. A replacement in perhaps a size eight or seven would be purchased.

3) The biopsy would be positive and I'd start my search for the Boobsy Twins as my prosthetic replacements.

I guess there could have been a fourth possibility—cancel the biopsy and arrange to take the next space shuttle to Mars. That didn't seem like a very plausible option, though.

On July 6 after the holiday weekend, I returned to work and received a call from my surgeon's secretary. My surgery had been scheduled for July 14 the following week. The fourteenth. Doesn't that ring a bell? It did for me. That was the one-year anniversary of my mastectomy. What does this mean? Should I start reserving operating room time for every July 14? Was this a sign that surgery was going to be an annual event?

I called Al at home and gave him the information about the date and time of the surgery. I waited until I got home to talk with my folks about the specifics. My mother sounded very distressed about the surgery being on the same day as the previous year's. It felt like an omen. I tried very hard not to think too much about it, but it wasn't easy. I decided to tell only a few people at work about it to avoid creating a panic. Didn't want rumors running rampant that I was about to go six feet under.

Since I was going to be receiving an IV sedative this time, I wanted to touch base with Dr. Pasternak, the medical director of the Outpatient Center. He's also an anesthesiologist. I connected up with him later in the week and told him I would be a patient in his neck of the woods the following week, and inquired as to who was scheduled that day as the "Sandman" of anesthesiology.

He told me he was one of the physicians scheduled that day, but would be happy to arrange for one of the female anesthesiologists to be with me for the procedure. I requested that he be present. He was someone I trusted and knew fairly well. Since I had a past history of respiratory problems from anesthetic agents, I preferred to deal with someone I knew and who knew me.

He was concerned that because I would be awake during the procedure, I might feel self-conscious about him seeing me topless. I assured him that my priority was my health status and not my modesty. Anyway, since my mastectomy the preceding summer I wasn't as shy as I used to be. Figuratively speaking, I was only half as shy.

Al once again had the unpleasant task of alerting our friends and other family members about this new development in our lives. Prayers were offered from everyone, and from all denominations of faith. It was very reassuring for me.

Al had a positive outlook about it, and felt that perhaps our luck had finally changed and this time the news would be good. I wanted to think as positively as he did, but found it harder this time. Nevertheless, I didn't lose my sense of humor, and we spent a lot of time joking about Betty possibly being replaced with a slightly smaller model, and that we would name twin prostheses if I needed them.

To further complicate my parents' lives, Dad was informed by his physician that his PSA level was high. He took a special blood test that can help detect abnormalities of the prostate gland. It is used as a marker for detecting prostate cancer. The results of his test meant he was also going to have a biopsy. His was scheduled two days after mine. I'm sure if my mother had her druthers, she would have gotten into the fantasy commercials for Calgon bath oil beads and simply said, "Calgon...Take me away," just like I wanted to do at this time the year before.

I was on vacation for two days before my surgery. I probably would have been better off working, but I took the time off anyway. We just didn't do the things we had originally planned to do during our vacation, like enjoy ourselves. The day before my surgery, several of my staff sent me a beautiful bouquet of flowers to wish me well. I also received several cards in the mail. That night I received a lot of phone calls from people offering prayers that my results would be good this time.

My surgery was scheduled for 12:15 on Wednesday. I asked my folks not to come, because they had just picked up my brother's family from the airport after midnight on Tuesday. They had flown in from Japan to again spend their vacation time with us. Laura was at my parents' farm with them. So it was just Al and me that day at the hospital.

It certainly felt like a *déjà vu* experience: being in the Same Day Surgery Suite, seeing the same faces I had seen one year before, putting on the hospital gown, feeling my heart race. Al waited in the waiting room while the nurses prepped me. He received a surprise visit from Marge and Scott. They gave him a card signed by many members of my department wishing me good things. Their timing was impeccable.

Once I was prepped, Al was allowed to rejoin me, and he stayed with me until it was time for me to go into surgery. He said he was fine but I could see the beginning of hives on his face. A female anesthesiologist came in to talk with me about my problem history with anesthesia, and said that she and another woman would be in the operating room with me. I was too nervous to ask about Dr. Pasternak, although I had seen him a few moments before. I suspected he preferred to have the female folks with me during the unveiling part of the preparation where the doctor has the patient topless for a few seconds until drapes are applied to the surgical site.

Charlie Yeo came to see me at this point, and was his usual cheerful and calming self. He asked me how I was doing, and I responded by saying I was as nervous as a whore in a church.

Within minutes I was being walked into the operating room. I

gave Al a big kiss, we exchanged "I love you's," and I was escorted into the chilly room where the deed was to be done once again.
The harder I tried not to shake, the more I shook. I felt embarrassed
about being so frightened, but was definitely more frightened than
embarrassed.

Silly as it may seem, I also had a fear once again that while
under the influence of drugs (conscious sedation) I'd talk and say
heaven knows what about whom. Maybe I'd feel some compelling
need to describe details about my sex life with my husband. Maybe
I'd be mean to those who were trying to take care of me and help
me in the operating room. I thought, "Oh, please God, don't let me
utter a word."

I had been with my father on several occasions when he was
awakening from general anesthesia, and he was always unpredictable about what he would do or say. On one occasion he was
very nasty and cursed a lot (to be specific, he wanted someone to
give him his teeth so he could, as he phrased it, bite his surgeon in
the rear end.) On another occasion while awakening from anesthesia, he turned into a Casanova, telling the recovery room nurse that
she had beautiful breasts and asking if he could touch them. I was
shocked! All of this behavior was very out of character for him.

Who knew what I might say or do under the influence of similar drugs? Remember, I would be seeing all of these faces again
and on a frequent basis, because I worked at the place where my
medical care was being provided.

Once I was on the operating room table, Charlie drew a circle
around the location of the lump. I was then placed in a horizontal
position on the table and strapped down. This is the point when the
patient realizes she is truly about to lose control of the situation and
must place her faith in the Lord and the health-care providers who
surround her. As Charlie exited the room, I heard the anesthesiologist say to go scrub up because my blood pressure was very high.
That was the last thing I remembered.

When I opened my eyes, I was in the recovery room and my
throat felt sore. I struggled to focus on the clock on the wall and

realized that several hours had passed. I knew then that I must have slept through the entire event. Al appeared. A nurse appeared. So did the anesthesiologist, director of nursing, medical director, and several other people, each inquiring how I felt. Each reassuring me that the procedure was over and I was okay now. True, I was phys-ically okay, but what was taken out of my breast?

Shortly after, Charlie appeared. Still calming and reassuring, he said he decided to put me under anesthesia because I was very upset during the procedure. But I didn't remember any of the pro-cedure. I asked if I had talked at all, and he wittily teased me and said, "Oh yes, you talked a whole lot." Then he smiled and shook his head no, saying I hadn't talked at all. I'll probably never really know if I did or not. For all I know, the entire surgical team that assisted Charlie now knew every position and technique my hus-band and I use in bed. Oh well, there's nothing I could do about it now. Hopefully if I did talk, I spoke about the weather (right—fat chance of that!).

Charlie said that the mass was fairly large, but the color of the tissue looked good and he felt hopeful this time. But he didn't want us to hang our hat on this preliminary news. Last year we thought everything was okay and got the unwanted surprise in the end. He told me to call him in five days to talk about the path report. Five days sounded like an eternity to me.

An hour or so later I was escorted out of the hospital via wheel-chair. Al picked me up at the door. Once home, I lay down to rest and put an ice bag on my bandages. Charlie had instructed me to wear my bra for a week around the clock to provide support to the surgical site. This meant that Betty would be sleeping in bed with Al and me. It was strange. I thought it would be uncomfortable having three pounds of silicone in bed with me but it wasn't. I found myself assuming sleeping positions I hadn't been able to use since my mastectomy. I hadn't even realized I'd developed differ-ent sleeping positions with my left arm until that moment. It made me feel melancholy for the flesh there prior to Betty's arrival.

Though the weekend was busy with my brother's family at

home with us from Japan, it was hard not to constantly think about what the verdict would be on Monday afternoon. On Friday I was at the hospital to be with my father during his prostate biopsy, and I stopped upstairs to see Charlie's secretary, Tracey. She advised me of his schedule for Monday and told me the best time to call would probably be after 1:30 p.m. I left a card for him. It was a personal note thanking him for getting me through this crisis to date, and telling him I would be back in touch with him on Monday afternoon for the verdict. The card, like most of the cards I send people, was a funny one. It had a cartoon drawing of a man and woman sitting in a ski lift chair. As they travel in it up the slope, they pass a sign that says, "PLEASE KEEP YOUR TIPS UP." The female skier, very well endowed, is sitting in the chair holding her boobs up with her hands. The man in the chair with her looks at her and says, "Excuse me, Miss, I believe the sign refers to one's skis!" Inside, the card said, "Seeing you is always an uplifting experience." I felt confident that Charlie would enjoy the card.

Monday finally arrived. When it did, I was in Reading, Pennsylvania, shopping with my sister-in-law at the outlet stores there. My energy level was low, but I was determined to shop with her. She was home from Japan only once a year, and this was her vacation time. It was my vacation time, too. I kept watching the clock. We were heading home and had reached Lancaster when the clock read 1:30 p.m. We stopped to eat lunch, so I called Charlie's office from a pay phone.

My heart was beating so fast I felt like it could have leaped out of my chest and run around the block without me. The restaurant was very noisy because of the people bustling in and out. I felt like turning into Miss Piggy and decking anyone who laughed or spoke loudly while walking by me. I thought this was how a maniac must feel right before he goes into a public place, takes out a semiautomatic gun, and blows away anything that moves. Where were those lunatics when you needed them? I certainly didn't want to kill anybody, but waving a large gun around might have quieted the room down, which was what I wanted.

I got a line through to Charlie's office and realized that the woman's voice on the other end was not that of his secretary. His secretary was not in at the time. The voice told me Dr. Yeo was still waiting for my path report results. Oh no. That would mean more waiting for me, too. She recommended I call back in an hour. I went back into the restaurant to join my sister-in-law and niece, and we ordered our food. I could hardly concentrate on the menu, much less eat what the waitress brought me. She could have served me a section of inner tube and I would probably have eaten it about the same way I ate the turkey platter I'd ordered. My brain was in oblivion, and my taste buds had traveled with my brain to keep it company.

By 2:30 we were nearing the completion of our meal. I excused myself and went out to the pay phone again. At last the verdict was in, and it was good news this time! No cancer! It was a benign mass of fibrocystic tissue. I didn't know who the pathologist was who dictated the report, but I loved him! I immediately called Al at home and told him the good news. He must have told me he loved me five times. I scampered back into the restaurant and went over to our table. "It's okay. It's benign." Then I broke into tears. Mary threw her arms around me and hugged me tightly. A crisis had passed once again. The dress rehearsal was over.

But how many more dress rehearsals would there be? None? Three? Ten? How can a breast cancer survivor distinguish a dress rehearsal from the real thing? There is no way. It starts with the first diagnosis, I suppose. Sure, some women may deal better with the fear of recurrence than others, but I'd wager money that there is no breast cancer patient who doesn't live with some degree of anxiety that the cancer will return. Return in the other breast, or return in some other part of the body. That's why it's important to maintain the support systems you have and use them whenever you need them. If you think that you're being a pain and bothering your friends or family, just remember the odds. One out of eight women develops breast cancer sometime during her lifetime. It is feared this number might be one in five in the year 2010.

While a friend or family member is helping you, they are also helping themselves. Helping themselves get acquainted with breast cancer and its treatments and pitfalls. There is a strong possibility that a person who is emotionally supporting you now is going to need your support in the future. During the first twelve months since my mastectomy, five of my friends have undergone breast biopsies and experienced the feeling of a dress rehearsal firsthand. One friend who underwent a breast biopsy was not as fortunate as the others. She became a breast cancer survivor club member and had her mastectomy only a few months after mine. She is our daughter's godmother. Little did she know that while she was providing me support and assistance through my crisis, she was actually helping to prepare herself for the same experience a few months later.

What can we do about this disease that has touched so many of us and so many of our friends? We can seek out the good things that come from undergoing such an experience. When you're going through it, it can be hard to find the good, but it's important to look within ourselves and seek it out. The roses do smell more fragrant now than in the past. Our family ties are more precious than we had realized before. Life is precious, and this experience reminds us not to waste it. That's why I became a nurse, I guess, so I could help people out during the troubled times in their lives. Help them get well again and get on with their business of living.

It's scary to think that approximately 180,000 women are diagnosed with breast cancer annually. Every three minutes a woman is newly diagnosed, and every eleven minutes, another woman dies of breast cancer. There have been nights I have lain in bed unable to sleep because so many things were on my mind. As I watched the clock slowly ticking one night, I realized that over a period of a little more than half an hour, three fellow club members somewhere in the United States had succumbed to this deadly disease. That's truly a startling thought.

That is why it's so important that we speak out—we who are club members and who are blessed to be among the survivors of the disease. We need to get involved with breast cancer support groups and help women who have been diagnosed after us to deal with the emotional roller coaster they are riding on. We need to learn how to deal with the anxiety and fear of possible recurrence from those who have been diagnosed and treated before us.

We need to promote breast cancer education in our community so more women will do breast self-exams and have annual physicals and annual mammograms.

This vigilance won't reduce the number of women diagnosed each year. It might actually increase the number. But it will reduce the numbers of deaths due to the disease. Early detection can usually guarantee a higher survival rate.

It's also important to get involved with legislation and promote and support bills in Congress directed toward research dollars going exclusively to breast cancer research, as well as bills that promote healthcare dollars being spent on mammography and treatment for women who would otherwise not receive any health-care.

Since my mastectomy surgery, I have been involved with local breast cancer support groups, including those available through the Internet. I feel I am helping others while benefiting myself, as well. When I reached my one-year anniversary as a breast cancer survivor, I was eligible to sign up as a Reach to Recovery volunteer. This gave me an opportunity to see patients who had undergone mastectomy surgery at Hopkins, discuss with them their emotions about their surgery, and help them through those early days of learning to live without a breast. It gives me a unique opportunity to blend my nursing skills with my mastectomy experience, while simultaneously working with health-care professionals I know and respect.

Reach to Recovery made some positive changes over the last several years or so, and now provides volunteers for visits before surgery as well as after. It is a pleasure to volunteer my evening hours in this way. I feel I am a stronger person for it.

My Avon representative, Judy Winebrenner, has given me little gift packs of Avon sample products to include in the mastectomy supplies I provide to women who have undergone a mastectomy like myself. I also supply women with literature from the American Cancer Society. Avon started a national breast cancer crusade campaign in September 1993, and now sells pink ribbon pins that are a symbol of breast cancer awareness. All the money raised by these sales is spent on breast cancer education.

I wear my pink ribbon pin with pride and am seldom without it on my clothing. I always make a point of wearing it when I am on my Reach to Recovery hospital visits. The sample items that Avon provided me as an R-to-R volunteer further exemplify the company's commitment to women. Avon wants all women to feel beautiful. During a medical crisis like breast cancer, when a woman may be doubting her femininity, Avon is there for her, too.

Chapter 19

The months passed quickly, and soon it was time for my next mammogram. That first real mammogram took place in June 1994. Why do I describe it as "real?" Because all the mammograms I'd had to date resulted from the development of symptoms that had required a mammogram to determine their cause. This mammogram was different. This time I had no lumps and no known signs of any problems. It had been a year since my previous mammogram; those films had been taken right before the lumpectomy on my remaining breast.

I felt nervous about having an X-ray taken this year because in the previous years I'd had my breast placed in the vise machine only when something was wrong. I guess you could say what I was feeling is what scientists call a "trident effect." If your association with something is always negative, then even if you would like it to be positive in a different situation, your stomach somehow remembers the negative association and makes you feel like you want to throw up.

Although I went into the mammography suite with butterflies in my stomach, I felt confident that this time I would be told what I had longed to hear: "Looks great! No abnormalities found."

But that wasn't what I was told. After having three different views taken, the technician told me that the radiologist had requested additional pictures because she "saw something." Oh, no. How could this be? After several more X-rays, I was taken to the sonogram room where the ultrasound was done. The objective of the ultrasound was to determine if the masses (yes, I said masses) were cysts (containing fluid) or tumors (solid in nature). Needle aspiration was attempted. After approximately one and a half hours, although I tried to keep my cool, I realized I was in the early stages of having another "experience."

Although I already had a routine appointment with my surgeon for a check-up in three weeks, the radiologist insisted that I call and get an appointment sooner. In the meantime, the radiologist very kindly made arrangements to dictate a report about my X-ray results and fax them to Charlie's office.

The anxiety that I and my family had felt before was once again present. It was hard to concentrate on work, but I knew that my best therapy would be to stay focused and occupied until I had more information about my situation. The radiology report looked ominous, however, so Al and I again discussed the serious possibility of "Betty Boob" officially getting a new roommate.

Al accompanied me to my appointment with Charlie Yeo. Al waited in the visitor's area while I got the verdict. No matter how hard I tried, I couldn't stop shaking. In a matter of moments, Charlie was with me and it again felt like *déjà vu*. He could see how nervous and upset I was. Fear of the unknown is truly the worst fear of all.

He reviewed the films with me and examined me. He said my body seemed prone to grow things in places that were already full grown, like my breasts. He told me it would be necessary to determine if these masses were benign or malignant, and that would require, at a minimum, another open biopsy.

Then we discussed what I felt was probably inevitable anyway—a second mastectomy. He spoke to me calmly and compassionately, realizing how emotionally difficult all of these experiences to date had been for me.

We discussed the positive aspects of choosing this option, and I told him I didn't want to keep coming to this office every summer to find out that my remaining breast had again grown something that needed removal. Being whittled away to nothing was not the route I wanted to take. I told him I agreed that the best option for me, whether the tumors were benign or malignant, was to "get Betty a new roommate." (I didn't have the courage to say the word mastectomy.)

I asked Charlie to talk to my husband. He very carefully asked me whether I wanted him to bring Al into the exam room, or if I wanted him to talk with Al alone. I pondered the question for about fifteen seconds, but it felt like five minutes. I chose to have them discuss the matter without me. Charlie left me to get dressed while he spoke with Al in a secluded part of the visitor's area. About five minutes later they came in together. Al told me the only thing that mattered to him was that I was with him, here on this earth, for as long as is feasibly possible, no matter what it took. Tears flowed down my face as if someone had turned on a faucet behind each eyeball. The reality of what was happening hit me hard.

Charlie asked us both to ponder our decision over the weekend and call on Monday to let him know if I still wanted to take this surgical route. We discussed it a lot over the weekend, and also talked with my parents and Laura about it. Everyone, including our daughter, to my surprise, felt that another mastectomy was the best option for me. Laura, now two years older than she was during my first mastectomy, told me she felt relieved because she had been worrying that the cancer might come back. She also thought that I looked great with Betty, and whoever I chose to be Betty's roommate would look equally good on me. Aren't children amazing?

The decision had been made. On Monday I called Charlie's office and confirmed a date for my surgery. It would take place June 27, two weeks from then. Once again, I implemented every support system I had. My parents, especially my mother, were coping much better this time. Maybe she was relieved that she could stop worrying about a recurrence of breast cancer. If the masses were cancerous they would be gone. If they were benign, we wouldn't have to worry about them turning into something worse later on or about my body producing more tumors. There would be virtually no breast tissue for them to grow in anymore.

It was very important for all of us to focus on the positives and not the negatives, and it was equally important to keep our sense of humor at all times. Prayers were being sent by many people. Mary, my roommate from nursing school, even arranged for special masses to be held for me in her church as well as in a convent on the

West Coast (and gee, I'm not even Catholic). My staff kicked into gear just as they had before, and I felt confident they would hold down the fort in my post-op absence.

On June 27, 1994, my second mastectomy was performed, and I went through my last stage of transformation. I wanted to wear a tassel on my nipple when I went into the operating room suite, but worried that the people assisting with the surgery, whom I didn't know personally, might find it too bizarre. Instead, I told my surgeon in front of everybody what I had planned to do but opted not to. Heaven only knows what those nice people thought of my telling Charlie of my strange plan when all of them were present.

To be safe, Charlie removed a few lymph nodes from my axillary area as well as from the chest wall. I was scheduled for discharge the following morning. Shortly before I was released Charlie came to check my incision. As he removed my binder and dressings to expose the incision, Al, as he had before, looked on with an expression of complete acceptance of my body.

Charlie said to me, "Your chest looks like my two-year-old daughter's chest. We've recently adopted a little girl from Russia. We feel that bringing her back to the States to live with us so she can be part of our family is like giving her the chance to be reborn. The case is the same for you, Lillie. You now look as if you've been reborn."

A more appropriate or thoughtful expression of caring and acceptance could not have been offered to me that day. It made me feel accepted. It made me feel special. It made me feel whole.

Nine days later I returned to see Charlie and have my hemovac drains pulled out and get information on my pathology results. The masses contained within the breast were in a precancerous state, and the lymph node results were negative. At last some good news! Al was thrilled, as were my parents and friends.

We immediately began adding to our list all the advantages of having the second surgery done: No more annual mammograms! No more worrying and fretting about the results! I could be whatever size I wanted to be now—I could look like Dolly Parton one day and Peter Pan the next!

There were things that would require time to adjust to. I worried about how this loss would affect our sex life. (Al didn't worry, but of course I did.) Al told me there is a proven theory that if you lose one of your senses (like your sense of sight or hearing), your other senses become more intensified. Therefore, he believed that if you lose one of your erotic zones, either you develop a new one some-place else or your remaining erotic zones become more intensified. He said it was his job to prove this hypothesis.

When I reached five weeks post-op, he took me away to the Pocono Mountains to prove his theory. I now call him Professor Shockney.

If it were possible to give him some type of honorary award I would. In my opinion, he should receive a Nobel Prize for proving that hypothesis!

Getting breast cancer was one of the worst experiences of my life. But in a way, it was also one of the best experiences, because of all I gained from it. When people ask me questions about breast cancer, I constantly reaffirm the positives.

Such as:

Question: *How has your marriage been since your mastec-tomies? How is your sex life?*

Answer: My marriage was good before, but now it's even stronger. I've always been happy with our sex life, but it, too, has also improved despite the loss of both of my breasts. If a woman's marriage is rocky, such an experience can push people to the edge. The final outcome is separation and divorce for some. It is doubtful that a husband leaves because a breast is gone. However, a series of misfortunes and differences of opinion are further complicated by breast surgery. My personal opinion about a husband who opts to leave is, "Good riddance to you. She deserved better all along."

Question: *How are your parents doing emotionally since all of this happened?*

Answer: They are doing well. Our family has always been close but now we are even closer than before. They are both very active in doing volunteer work to raise funds to support cancer screening, education, awareness, and research, with a special focus on helping people in the community where they live. My mother and I also cofounded a nonprofit organization in 1995 called Mothers Supporting Daughters with Breast Cancer. (See Chapter 21 for details.)

Question: *How is your daughter?*
Answer: She couldn't be better. She is one of my best supporters and has educated other teenagers like herself about my experience. (She is no longer worried about being small-breasted, having graduated this past summer to a 36D bra!) I am constantly amazed at how resilient children can be. If we listen closely to what they have to say, we can benefit from their wisdom. You will find that a five-year-old watching her grandmother soak in the tub is perfectly accepting of her grandmother's appearance, and is completely unconcerned that she has one breast instead of two. That's because children haven't lost sight of what unconditional love is.

Question: *What other reasons do you have for considering breast cancer a positive experience?*
Answer: I've met people who, under normal circumstances, I never would have met. I've had the opportunity to spend time with breast cancer survivors who became club members after me, and to help them through difficult moments that can only be shared and conquered with the help of another club member. I've felt the exhilaration of going to the Susan G. Komen Race for the Cure breast cancer events, where I am physically surrounded by thousands of other club members and their supporters. I have been given the opportunity to speak to large and small groups, such as mastectomy support groups, volunteers who work with cancer patients, and organizations holding fund-raisers for cancer research and awareness. With each presentation I feel rejuvenated,

just like the Energizer Bunny.

Question: *Did you decide to name your other prosthesis after your second mastectomy?*
Answer: Yes! Betty's roommate is named Bobbie (Bobbie Sue, to be precise).

Question: *Do you think you will always do volunteer work for the Reach to Recovery Program?*
Answer: Yes, I certainly hope so. I want to see the program continue to evolve to meet the special needs of women with breast cancer. With hospitalization lengths of stay now averaging less than twenty-four hours for mastectomy surgery, we need to develop additional mechanisms to support breast cancer patients after surgery. One thing I have noticed about the new "club members" I visit at the hospital is their sense of bonding with me, particularly once I tell them I have opted not to have reconstruction done. They look at my chest and smile. They aren't smiling because they want to be socially polite to Betty and Bobbie Sue. They smile, I think, because they realize I am on the same playing field they are. They are lying in a hospital bed without a breast, or possibly without either breast, and they realize I am just like they are, except farther along in my recovery. I am a walking example that there is life, love, joy, and happiness after breast cancer, and that reconstruction isn't a requirement to achieve happiness—it is only one option out of many.

Question: *Where do you see cancer research going now?*
Answer: We are on the brink of a new era of research methodology. In the past, treatments for cancer have focused on what Dr. Susan Love calls the "slash, poison, and burn" methods. Slash—cut the cancer out. Poison—use chemotherapy to destroy it. Burn—use radiation to kill it. Now we are entering a biological era. Gene identification. Antibody therapy. Vaccines. Rather than using traditional ways of treating cancer, scientists are looking at

developing ways to help the body repair the cells that have mutated and are on a transformation into cancer cells. (Few people realize that a cancer cell is one of your own cells that has mutated and "gone bad.")

Question: *What role do you want to play in the future regarding breast cancer treatment?*

Answer: I want to be and stay wherever the action is! I want to help the organizations committed to prevention. I want to be involved with researchers who are developing ways to provide early detection for premenopausal women, since conventional mammography often doesn't get all tumors, especially for women under age forty. I want to facilitate ways in which the care and treatment provided to women with breast cancer are the very best they can be, so they meet the patient's expectations regarding physical, psychological, cultural, and spiritual needs.

One group of people often left to fend for themselves emotionally are mothers of women with breast cancer. My mother and I have started a national nonprofit organization for them called "Mothers Supporting Daughters with Breast Cancer." It is devastating for a mother to see her daughter go through such an experience, and many mothers feel guilty if they have had breast cancer, too. Those who have not been touched by this villain themselves wish it was happening to them rather than to their daughters. These women need special support from one another, and from others who have weathered the storm before them. Since March 1995, we have helped more than 12,000 sets of mothers and daughters. It is truly a gratifying experience to reach out and support these women who are following in our footsteps.

Having a clinical background, being a breast cancer survivor, and having expertise in the field of quality of care measurements places me in a unique situation. I have a lot to offer to those organizations looking to improve the quality of care and services provided to women with breast cancer and their families. I am compelled to do so, too.

MAKING CHANGES IN MY LIFE

Once anyone has been touched by breast cancer, her life is different. Mine is, and for the better. I began doing volunteer work for the Johns Hopkins Breast Center in 1994, spending about twenty hours a week after regular working hours and on weekends. Having the opportunity to help support new club members became increasingly important to me. I also assisted with various performance improvement initiatives that the faculty and nursing staff worked on, each designed to improve patient care and make the treatment of breast cancer less traumatic for future patients.

My husband said whenever I stayed late at the hospital, he could tell whether I'd been working on something related to my job or working voluntarily on breast cancer projects. He said, "No matter how late it is or how tired you might be, when you have stayed late to work with breast cancer patients or with the Breast Center team, you walk with a bounce. You are energized rather than fatigued." He was right. And my need to do it more and more grew steadily.

In July 1997 I was given the wonderful opportunity to transfer the Johns Hopkins Breast Center into a new position called director of education and outreach. In this role I am responsible for our performance improvement initiatives, each designed to improve patient care. I also oversee our website, educational programs, outreach efforts, and have a team of more than seventy-one breast cancer survivor volunteers, each one having been diagnosed and treated at Johns Hopkins in the past for breast cancer. These special people provide many services to our patients.

A critical service they provide is one-on-one support for newly diagnosed patients. We give patients the option of being matched with a survivor volunteer based on her age, stage of disease, anticipated treatment plan, and other factors important in making the match work well.

One patient said to me, "Oh, I see. You are assigning me a bosom buddy." I suppose she was right! The volunteer stays connected with the patient for as long as the patient wishes, which usually is all the way through to the end of treatment. For some patients, that can be more than a year of time.

Our survivor volunteers also help with educating others in their local communities about breast cancer awareness, promoting breast self-exams and mammography, attending health fairs with us, and other breast cancer-related items.

As a special monthly project, we also make gift baskets for our patients. The patient receives the gift basket in the recovery room when she awakens from surgery. It contains "comfort items," all of which have been donated. These include such items as aromatherapy, potpourri, books of women's poetry, gift certificates for a facial or a pedicure, Avon products, herbal tea, cosmetics, bubble bath, and many other items—each intended to help her hold tight to her femininity, which has been threatened by the surgery she has had that day.

I give about thirty speeches a year now and travel all over the country to deliver various messages. Some are serious ones, focusing on breast cancer, its possible causes, and strategies for new treatments and prevention. My favorite talk, however, comes from this book—my personal experiences with breast cancer and how I have used humor as one of the weapons to help me become a survivor. Many more funny stories have occurred in the last few years that could be put to paper, and perhaps at some point I'll write another book and include them. What is most fun is that funny things continue to happen, and that's because I seek out the humor in what could be an embarrassing or depressing situation.

I had the opportunity to be the plenary speaker for a special event at Hopkins called "A Woman's Journey." My speech was an abbreviated version of a longer talk that I give, which includes stories about Miss Bertha, and Laura, our daughter, and my own personal experiences with breast cancer as a patient and supporter of others who end up wearing my bra. More than 1,200 women were in the audience for that special event, and it was a thrill to receive a standing ovation at the close of my talk. It doesn't matter if the audiences is large, like that one, or a handful of people—it gives me joy to share my story and hopefully inspire others to look at breast cancer differently in the future.

There is little doubt in my mind that I was meant to get breast cancer. It is rare that we learn while here on this earth why bad things happen to us, but I was blessed with being given the answer early on. That answer is so I can provide support to other club members who follow behind me. It is so I can effect change in traditional treatment and think out of the box and develop ways that breast cancer treatment will be easier for women diagnosed in the future.

Improvements in the surgical treatment for breast cancer that have been achieved at Hopkins since my second mastectomy are amazing and something that all of the faculty and staff can take great pride in. Women awaken in the recovery room nausea-free and pain-free and feel the sensation of being surgically transformed from a victim into a survivor. It is now a day of celebration and not a day of sadness.

Dr. William Dooley, the medical director of the Breast Center and a surgical oncologist who is truly one of the most dedicated people I've ever known, is to be commended for making this possible. Not a day goes by that we don't take a few moments to talk about what we can do as a team to make the best we've achieved at Hopkins even better. We are constantly striving to find a cure, too. Research is so important and must not end or be curtailed until this is achieved.

So when someone says to me, "Gee, I guess if you had your druthers you'd wish this never happened to you, right? Don't you wish your breasts were back?" I can say "no" confidently, because what I've gained in exchange for this experience is immeasurable for the joy it has provided.

Do I miss my breasts? Sure. But I don't dwell on that. I've exchanged them for another chance at life. A chance at life filled with opportunities to help others in extraordinary ways that was not possible prior to having breast cancer myself. Though I felt I was a good nurse, I now realize that having personally experienced this disease makes me a better nurse, a better person.

A woman asked me not long ago, "Don't you get upset when you get in the shower and look down and see that your breasts are gone?" I responded by saying, "I look down and see that the cancer is gone." My glass is half full, not half empty. My surgeries transformed me from a victim into a breast cancer survivor. What I gained far exceeds that which I lost, though what I lost was precious to me. I look at life as a gift and don't take it for granted anymore.

I now have the special opportunity to combine my nursing skills, personal breast cancer experiences, and expertise in the area of quality measurement and improvement to make things better for women diagnosed after me. What a life. I've already testified on Capitol Hill, been on television more than thirty times, given more than two hundred talks across the country, and written numerous articles about breast cancer. In October 1998 I was the recipient of a national award for a document I wrote called "Breast Cancer: Making the Right Choices for You." The document serves as a guide to help newly diagnosed women ensure that they are in good hands when proceeding with treatment of this disease. This document can be found in Appendix A (page 189) as well as on the Johns Hopkins Breast Center website (www.med.jhu.edu/breastcenter/) and on the Intelihealth website (www.intelihealth.com).

I am very knowledgeable now about breast cancer and its treatment, and I strive to learn more every day. My knowledge far exceeds what I knew when I underwent my own treatment. This aids me in being able to help and advise others, which is important to me now. If I make the experience easier for just one club member undergoing treatment now, or effect change for improvements in the future, then I have been successful. If I hadn't gotten breast cancer I would have missed out on so much and not been afforded the opportunity to meet so many people who are special in my life—so many club members and their families who are now part of my life and my future. *Shape* magazine and the National Race for the Cure honored me in June 1999 with their national award called "Circle of Life" in recognition of my personal and professional work in the field of breast cancer. Also in 1999, Intel named me an "Internet Health Hero."

A lady asked me, "Do you still have cleavage now that both of your breasts are gone?" I repeated to her one of my favorite sayings: "My doctor surgically removed my 'cleav' and left me with my 'age'—with the intent that I grow old." Each year that I do grow older, I thank God for the opportunities bestowed upon me as result of this experience.

I am a believer in fate and think things happen to us for a reason. Prior to July 1992, I didn't know just how precious life is. I wasn't aware of my own mortality. Now I've looked Death in the face. When he smiled at me and said "not yet," I began to value each day. The sunset is gorgeous even when it's raining.

I purchased a postcard for myself as a reminder of how women are viewed in society. It's a photograph of a young girl, about age ten, standing on a beach with a woman about age thirty. This woman is probably the girl's mother, but could have been an aunt or a neighbor, even an older sister. They are both wearing T-shirts and have their eyes closed. They stand with their chests proudly sticking out as they arch their necks back to drink in the sunshine, surf, and salt air. The T-shirt on the child says, "Watch this space." This photo means so many things to me, especially the knowledge of how important breasts are in our society, and the realization that every girl wants to "watch this space" grow normally and still be attached to her when she dies of old age. We need to encourage and facilitate more watchers to be doers. What I mean is, there are those who *say* they want to help in the fight against breast cancer and there are those who *do* something to help with the fight. I am a doer. I want to see more doers. If you are a watcher, become a doer; if you are already a doer, thank you. Together, as a united force, we *can* do it—we can prevent breast cancer.

I am now a regular speaker for various associations, organizations, and fund-raising events for cancer, and I enjoy speaking very much. My goal is to be like the Maytag repairman. I'm sure you've all seen the commercials on television. He sits in his office all day long, alone and very bored, waiting for the phone to ring. If the phone were to ring, it would mean someone needed his expert assistance in repairing a Maytag washing machine. But in the commercial, the Maytag repairman's phone never rings.

I receive several calls a week from various people who need to talk about breast cancer. It might be someone who needs me to see a patient in the hospital, or it might be a friend who knows someone who has just been diagnosed with breast cancer and is seeking advice on treatment or just information about the disease.

I want to be like the Maytag repairman. I want no one out there to need my help and support. I want to see breast cancer become a part of medical history for my future grandchildren and great-grandchildren to read about in textbooks, not know about from personal experience. When the phones stop ringing across the country that are currently linked to breast cancer support groups, coalition organizations, breast cancer treatment centers, cancer associations, Reach to Recovery, and other breast cancer-related programs, we'll all be able to sleep better at night knowing that this disease has finally been stopped dead in its tracks. Mothers, daughters, granddaughters, spouses, and friends of the future will sleep better, too.

I have a lot of degrees behind my name, and each took a lot of blood, sweat, and tears to earn. But one degree I've earned doesn't appear on my business cards like the others do. It's the one I take the greatest pride in achieving and requires the most CEUs (continuing education units) to maintain. It is my "CS" degree—my Cancer Survivor degree. If you have this degree and read this book for the purpose of getting to know other club members better, you know how hard it is to get this degree. If you read my story because you are a nurse or other health-care professional seeking insight into the thoughts and feelings of breast cancer patients, I want you to remember this: The next time you are looking into the eyes of a woman with breast cancer, know that the next pair of victim's eyes you look into might be your own.

If you are interested in having me give a presentation at a breast cancer support organization or nursing association meeting, please let me know. I welcome the opportunity to share my story. It is one of the most positive aspects of having become a club member, and I do it often. Numerous organizations have obtained copies of my book directly from the publisher and sell it as a fund-raiser to support their work. If you want to reach me for this purpose, or for any other reason, please write to me at this address:

Lillie Shockney, RN, BS, MAS
307 Bond Avenue
Reisterstown, MD 21136-1405

Chapter 20
The Parents' Chapter

Dad's Story

It was rather strange when our daughter, Lillie, called and asked if I would write a little bit about being a parent of a cancer victim. Since I consider myself a rough and tough farmer, it is very difficult to talk about the things I feel, or put them into print. If you are the person diagnosed with cancer, bear with me as I share my thoughts for a few pages.

I was watching a program on TV when our daughter called, and I borrow the title from the movie I was watching: *The Day the Bubble Burst*. The movie was the story of the 1929 market crash.

Our family started out as very poor farmers, always struggling to make ends meet. After finally breaking through, I thought we had it all. We had political power, we had prestige in the community, and we were financially comfortable—able to buy the things we needed, at least anything we thought we needed.

The day the bubble burst, I was in the shop a hundred feet away from the house. I heard a noise. I came in thinking that my wife was laughing, which was very unusual, but soon realized that she was crying. She had broken down, I think for the first time in her life. Finally, I got her quieted down enough to hear that Lillie had called and said it was cancer. Many questions immediately came to my mind. Have I contributed to it? Why my family? Why my child? Why not me? I crawled back in my big green glass-enclosed monster—on the farm tractor by myself so I could think. I thought of everything, I suppose. I thought how when Lillie was growing up she was fortunate, or unfortunate perhaps, to be born to two workaholic parents. I did not take the time when she was growing up to be with her as I should have. I was busy keeping the wolf from our door and attempting to make a comfortable future for us.

We purchased a 4-H calf for her and, darn the luck, it turned out to be a sterile one. She then got into 4-H speaking and was very good at it, but sometimes not being in the clique of people running the show in the State 4-H contest caused those not as deserving to be State winners. However, the 4-H speaking experiences served her well throughout her life, as we know.

She was very subtle at getting what she wanted. She always worked for what she wanted and needed. I remember our house was a rather rough-looking old farmhouse back then. Lillie's subtle way of waking up Dad was to go in the yard and use her talents as an artist to paint our house. When I finally saw the house in a picture, I knew it was time to fix up the place. She said that I had fixed up the outbuildings and bought new machinery, so she went on a binge to rebuild the house and make things look better. This was her way of getting what she needed, and what she knew her mother wanted.

I can relate many, many stories about her compassion. How she touched people when she was growing up. When I had a serious chemical burn, she would drive home fifty miles one way, after being in class all day, to give my injury a Betadine scrub so my leg wouldn't get infected and scar. She worked for Dr. Kaufman in Rock Hall when she finished nursing school. Since then, I have heard many people talk about how compassionate she is. They said they couldn't have made it without her. Compassion is her trademark. Doing for others and not asking for anything in return.

Why does cancer occur in this type of person? The only reason I can give is that perhaps by having cancer, Lillie will be able to educate and help many, many others, including parents and children.

When you hear the word CANCER for your daughter, and you have a beautiful granddaughter, your thoughts leave the other members of your family and focus on them. You wonder what will happen to your granddaughter. Who will raise her? Where will she go to school? What will she miss out on? After only a day of thinking about these things, I was able to say to my wife with total conviction, "Don't worry. Lil will make it." Since the beginning of this crisis, I've said that Lil would see her child raised and educated. A year later, we know she will.

As a father, I have gone back over the farming chores we had for our children while they were growing up. The chemicals we used on the farm had no warnings about their danger. We sprayed the spittle bugs on the hay with a chemical. The flies in the barn were sprayed with DDT. There were no restrictions and no guidance as to the use of these chemicals. If a little would work, you put on more. Airplanes covered the cornfields with Toxiphene and other related chemicals for cutworm. We handled chemicals of all kinds, and used them in the production of corn, soybeans, hay, and cattle. I look back, wondering if some of these chemicals were the culprit. We live near Aberdeen, which was a proving ground, and Edgewood, which was a proving ground for chemicals. I wonder if that was the source of Lillie's cancer.

When she was a child, did the ships coming down the Bay pumping out their bilges contribute to it? Or is this just Mother Nature and God saying, "Well, we really need to wake up some people, and this is how we're gonna do it." I think I can say, without contradiction, that this experience has changed our lives.

I know Lillie is one of the most compassionate people I have ever known, but if there was a way for her to become more compassionate, I think this was it. Wherever I've had any problems, or had to go to the hospital for something, her hand on my shoulder or her standing by my bed had a more tranquilizing effect than any medicine could have. Her touch sends a peaceful medicine into your body. She and I had a close relationship. When we see each other, we either hold hands or put our arms around each other, and it's not necessary to say anything. We know what the other is thinking.

As I look back at Lillie and her experience with cancer, I realize that maybe something made her plan in advance for a battle she didn't yet know she was going to fight. She had a good husband, a good job, and many friends. I think this was her salvation. The friends she made seemed to unite in prayer in best wishes for her. I suppose prayer was one of the strongest things to help her through, but the laughter and happiness she displayed to other people while concealing her own fears is another big part of it. She knows how to laugh; she knows how to enjoy life; she knows how to be compassionate with other people. These attributes have been her salvation.

In November 1998, I received the dreaded news that many men receive—cancer of the prostate. My reaction was not as controlled as I thought it should have been for the first few days. Then I said, "If Lillie can beat cancer twice, I can beat it once!"

We shared many, many loud laughs (the miracle cure) as I went through bone scans, biopsies, and other related studies. Lillie, her mother, and I shared many of our most intimate experiences. Several times, while in a conference with the doctor, Lillie would break all of us up when she could tell the doctor we were two older people who still acted like lovesick teenagers, especially when I exclaimed, "My goodness! Don't take it away from us!"

Once again she showed her compassion from the time treatments began until they were completed two months later. Because of her faith and her sense of humor that she shared with me and the technicians, I was able to drive myself 230 miles each day for the thirty-nine treatments.

If you are the recipient of news that you have cancer, don't try to blame yourself. Don't try to blame everyone else. Don't ask "why me?" If any advice should be followed, it is this: Take a big yellow pad. Write down the good things that have happened in your life; then write down the bad. If you are supporting a loved one with cancer be there when you are needed, but have the good sense to let the person have time to themselves sometimes. Take life one day at a time, and realize that money won't buy everything. Understand that friends, prayers, and memories of good times, good laughter, and a close relationship with your family will help the doctors and the good hospitals to restore you to good health. Now, as a cancer survivor myself, I can truly say that having experienced cancer makes you a better friend and a more helpful person—one who has the outlook of making the most of each day that God gives to us.

Mom's Story

There are lyrics to a song from a few decades ago that say: "It's what you do with what you've got and never mind how much you've got. It's what you do with what you've got that pays off in the end." Those words could have been written about us. In 1946 when we were married, we had little money but we dreamed of better things. Fortunately, we had the energy to make some of our dreams pan out.

God blessed us with two "whole" children who brought us tremendous joy. They were a month short of three years apart, which some of our friends said was the worst thing that could happen. Well, we proved them wrong on that score, and on many others. It turned out, in my mind anyway, to be perfect timing. The older one, our son, thought it was wonderful to have a little sister. Being a take-charge type, he immediately assigned himself as her protector.

As you've learned in earlier chapters, our daughter seemed to be plagued with various ailments but appeared to be the healthier child. Fortunately, none of her unusual health concerns seemed to deter her from accomplishing fantastic things at very early ages. Being on a farm afforded both of our children on-the-scene education that takes years for city children to learn. It really gave them a leg up on other students.

At the age of three, our daughter began performing before audiences, singing songs we learned together; songs that were long and difficult even for adults to learn. She never had stage fright or knew what being bashful meant. It was second nature to her, almost like breathing. I really believe that music was the thread that bound the family together. We always felt the need to turn to it when things were going sour, and it helped us see our way clear to surviving the difficulty at hand.

There have been a number of times in my life when I've said, "If I can live through this mess, I can live through anything." As I look back at some of the things I called a "crisis," it almost makes me laugh. Some of them were child's play in comparison to the things waiting around the corner in later years. It sort of reminds me of the progress children make. In the early stages, learning to walk is the biggest event of their lives. Later it might be the challenge of riding a two-wheeler. Sometimes it might be learning how to produce what a teacher expects of you, even though you dislike the format he or she insists the term paper must comply with.

When our school board changed the district boundary lines for students who attended Chestertown High School and Rock Hall High School, which made it necessary for our children to change schools even though we had not moved, I was ready to put up my fists and do battle. These were rival schools ever since they had been established. Our son was about to enter his senior year, so he was permitted to complete his last year in Chestertown if we provided transportation. However, our daughter was entering the ninth grade, so there was no way for her continue to attend the Chestertown school. Before this decision was made, the two had worked out a wonderful plan. He would play basketball and she would be a cheerleader. Now that he could drive, they could attend games together and come home in our car. They were crushed to learn that their plans would never become a reality.

So my famous statement came forth again: "If I can live through this mess, I can live through anything." The rival schools played games on different nights, of course, except when they played each other. We would attend "home" games, sitting on one side for the first half to cheer one team on, and sitting on the other side for the second half to cheer the other team on. I thought that was one of the most difficult times of my life, but I didn't know what was waiting around the corner. At this stage, I am talking about youngsters who were fourteen and seventeen years old.

We survived. Many years have passed since the rival schools

year, and many other crises have developed. Each time I came forth with my famous statement, I wondered if I would be ready for the next challenge with my name on it. I began to adjust better, or at least I thought I did. Many times folks didn't understand that my ability to cope with these crushing blows was not due to insensitivity. It was strength to see a situation through to the end without folding. It was holding on in spite of adversity.

We've had hailstorms that destroyed corn crops, a fire that wiped us out of the dairy business, and droughts that made us wonder why we put so much blood, sweat, and tears into the farming business. All of these things seemed to swat us down, but we always returned to do battle another day. Although these situations make one feel somewhat helpless, the hope of doing better next time was never destroyed.

My husband's mother once said that when a child is born, you worry about it until either you or it dies. She was correct in making that statement. I thought I could handle nearly anything that came my way. Through level-headedness and prayer, many trying things were overcome. Then we got a call from our daughter, a delightful, bubbly young woman with wit so sharp that one wondered why she didn't have a daily newspaper column, or some other way to share it with others who needed a laugh to survive the day. When I heard her say she was going for a mammogram, I knew something was very wrong.

All of the articles I have read indicated that a woman should begin annual mammograms when she turns forty. She was only thirty-eight, so I knew she wouldn't do this unless she thought there was a real need for it. She confessed that four years earlier she had a mammogram done because there was a cyst in her right breast. It was drained and everything was fine. I wondered how much more had occurred that she had not wanted to worry us with. Sure enough, the mammogram showed another cyst in her breast, but she was assured that it could be drained as before. The film of the other breast was checked, and there was something suspicious about it. This was the breast that had given no indication of anything wrong.

The waiting period between the time we knew that something was suspicious and when the pathology report from the biopsy was due was an eternity. Each day when Lillie returned from work, I called to find out what she knew. Each day, she still had heard nothing. I prayed that everything was all right. Finally, when I called one day there was a hesitation in her voice. She quietly said, "It wasn't what we wanted." I knew this was a new crisis. I kept my composure until I hung up the phone. At that moment, I felt as though someone had just told me Lillie was dead and I should prepare for a funeral in two days. I know that sounds very strange, particularly from a person who had always been able to stay together regardless of what was going on. But this time I felt the wrong generation had been attacked. It was not her turn. I could handle it much better myself. Mothers can heal themselves easier than having their loved ones in pain.

I began crying and sobbing as though she was already gone. What am I going to do to help her now? How am I going to help our granddaughter? How am I going to help my husband, her father, who believes that she can almost walk on water? When my husband came into the house and found me weeping, he surmised what was wrong. All I had to say was I had heard from Lillie. He later said it was the first time in the fifty years we had known each other that he saw me go to pieces immediately upon hearing bad news. Usually I held up until a crisis was over before I showed the effects of it.

"I can't stand it," I repeated again and again. "There is nothing fair about this. She doesn't smoke or drink. All she is guilty of is working too hard. Why are energetic people punished like this? I could handle this much better if it happened to me instead." I went on and on. He tried to comfort me, but there was little he could do when he felt as bad as I did. It is the most helpless feeling one can experience. Your child is told she has cancer, and there is no magic wand to make it disappear. It isn't just a bad dream that you will wake up from. There is no way to escape.

There were several things I was working on at that time, and as I was making notes about them I was constantly using the wrong date. I was stuck in May, it seemed. That was prior to the announcement that cancer had found another fertile spot to grow. I suppose I wanted time to reverse, so I wouldn't know we had a new crisis on our hands. The brain works in strange ways. I completely forgot my sister's wedding anniversary and her husband's birthday. They came and went in July, but I was still catching myself dating things in May.

Nothing seemed to be going right for me. Fortunately, I didn't have what I used to call "a real job" away from home. The work I do now is freelance or keeping the farm books, so my use of the wrong month could be corrected without harm. I functioned like a robot. Many things were done by rote. Some things weren't done at all. Some things that seemed very important in the past no longer had meaning or value. I called my friends, who were members of various churches, and asked that our daughter be placed on their prayer lists. We had people praying all over the county and in other parts of Maryland, the District of Columbia, Colorado, even half-way around the world (since our son and his family were stationed in Japan).

After the mastectomy was completed, there was another waiting period. I was failing in the section marked "patience." I felt as though I wanted to find the people in the labs where the testing was done to make sure they were doing their jobs properly. The family accuses me of always wanting to have things done properly anyway. Why not? That's what a person is paid to do. I also wanted the folks in the labs to get moving before I was totally crazed with concern about the whole thing. Fortunately, I wasn't denying this was serious, even though I wanted the clock to turn back to a time when everyone was well, or at least when we thought everyone was. I just wanted answers and I wanted them pronto, not later.

As the days dragged on friends inquired about our daughter each time I ran into them—on the street, in the grocery store, anywhere. Each time I spoke with them I found myself getting teary-eyed and had to apologize for showing such emotion. One day, however, when a family acquaintance asked about her, the tears welled up. He said quickly, "Oh, I'm sorry that I asked. Please excuse me." I knew then that I had to get ahold of myself. The last thing I wanted was to turn off folks who were genuinely interested. I had a firm talk with myself and made it very clear that I could do better. As luck would have it, I saw the same man that evening at a meeting and thanked him for making me realize I could control my inner feelings, particularly when folks who inquire are genuinely interested in Lillie's health. Fortunately, the lymph node tests were negative, so we felt the tide finally had turned in our favor. Now it was really time to give thanks for our blessings.

Exactly one year later (June 1993) Lillie's health was about to be challenged for a second time. She said it was nothing to worry about because the decision was a lumpectomy. A parent worries anyway. This time it was less stressful, particularly when the lab report indicated this mass was benign. All of us breathed easier. About a third of that breast was taken, so a new prosthesis for the left side was required to have both sides equal. This was a small item compared to the event in 1992.

I made another rash statement during this episode. I said I realized how difficult it was for me to handle stress during her mastectomy the year before. Then I foolishly remarked that we had learned so much from that experience and even though I hoped it never would happen again, I knew that I could handle it better if it did.

The next occasion for Lillie to have a mammogram was the summer of 1994. We could barely stand it when she announced I would have another chance to show everyone how well I could do as the mother of a breast cancer victim. Could this really be happening again? Yes, we were back on our knees praying for her to get through another major surgery—her second mastectomy.

Her father and I made the trek to the Johns Hopkins Hospital again and waited for the surgeon to tell us that her chances for survival were excellent. Fortunately, during the months that had passed since her first mastectomy, many improvements had been made in the medications and the anesthesia administered. As a result, she did not experience the terrible nausea that was part of the surgery two years before. This not only made Lillie more comfortable, it also was a big boost to the family members around her. All of us felt this was much easier than before. Of course, by this time we were "conditioned" for the surgery compared to the first time. We knew what to expect, or at least we thought we did.

From the first time when Lillie's life had been threatened with breast cancer until after the third surgery, all three summers I kept saying there should be an organization to help a mother emotionally so she can get through this ordeal. Again and again I harped on this subject. Lillie had checked everywhere (hospitals, cancer clinics, the Internet) and told me there weren't any in the whole country.

As the last resort, she posted a note on a message board on the Internet asking if anyone knew of an organization that offers emotional assistance for mothers whose daughters had been diagnosed with breast cancer. The next day she received 115 e-mail responses. No one knew of such an organization, but asked her to let them know if she found one. They indicated there were many mothers in need of an organization for that purpose.

Later, Lillie phoned me. "Mom," she said, "I am still looking for an organization to help the mothers of breast cancer victims. Now I have an idea! There is none, so we have to do it." I was astonished! When I asked Lillie what she meant, she said that, as a family, we had experienced three summers of trying to cope with this awful stuff. As a result, she said, I would know exactly how other mothers felt.

When I asked her how we would handle this, a brand new project in my life, she felt we could put on paper some of the ideas we found helpful and have a "handbook" a mother could use to give her the help she needed to see her daughter through this experience.

We did just that and the rest is now history. In March 1995 we held our organizational meeting, declaring the name of a new organization in the cancer world. It would be known as Mothers

Supporting Daughters with Breast Cancer (MSDBC). By sending letters to women's magazines, we began receiving requests from mothers who were going through the same trauma that I had known when I first learned Lillie was a cancer victim. We applied for—and after several months received—our nonprofit status.

During these years that have followed, we have assisted more than we can count. Because our literature goes to cancer centers and hospitals as well as to individuals, we do not know how many people we have helped. We have a policy that we will send our packet of literature to anyone requesting it, anywhere in the world. As a result of our websites, we receive requests from families, individuals, and professionals all over the globe.

Anyone wishing to reach us may do so by e-mail:
msdbc@dmv.com
or: Lilliepie@aol.com
Currently we have two Web sites:
www.mothersdaughters.com
www.azstarnet.com/~pud/msdbc/

I believe God has spared all of us for a reason. We now need to continue to be crusaders who tell others that there is life after cancer; that there is life after mastectomy; that parents can be supportive to each other as well as to the family member who is the cancer survivor. Now I can say that Lillie has opted to lose her body parts in order to save her life. She has taught all of us many lessons throughout the years, but making us realize how precious life can be is probably the most important lesson of all.

Chapter 21

HELPFUL HINTS FOR BREAST CANCER PATIENTS, THEIR FAMILIES, AND CONCERNED FRIENDS

This chapter is designed to be a resource for women who have been diagnosed with breast cancer. It contains information for the patient, as well as suggestions for family members and friends who will be involved in her treatment and recovery. Based on your individual situation you may choose not to utilize all sections of this chapter. It is here merely as a reference for you.

HELP HER STAY FEELING FEMININE

When a woman is confronted with the news that she is going to lose her breasts, it is not uncommon that fearing a loss of femininity accompanies fear of death from cancer. Breasts have long been a symbol of womanhood. The loss of a breast can cause a woman to doubt her attractiveness and make her fear she will be considered less of a woman.

Here are some suggestions for small gifts that can help to enhance a woman's femininity and promote a more positive self-image. For those of you on a tight budget, these items can be purchased in most cosmetic centers, Rite Aid Pharmacies, Wal Mart, and other similar chain stores at very reasonable prices. Your Avon representative is also an excellent person to purchase these types of items from. It's particularly nice to purchase small containers of these items. You might consider the "one-time-use" samplers that usually cost less than a dollar. Items such as a facial mask come in a flat one-time-use pouch and can be mailed in an envelope with a greeting card.

• Bubble bath—sizes range from tiny travel size plastic bottles to jumbo economy size.

• Facial mask—some favorites are the new anti-stress masks.

• Sachets for her lingerie drawer—some come in flat envelopes; others are in satin or mesh netting.

• Fragrance soaps.

• Small soft pillows—for use after surgery to support the affected arm.

• Book of verses about womanhood or the special friendship shared among women.

• Bookmarks—these can be especially fun! They range from the inspirational to photos of naked men (which could also be called "inspirational"). You can write a special note on the back to her as well.

• Jewelry—this could be a small locket or perhaps a charm for a charm bracelet or necklace.

• Romance novel.

• A gift certificate for a facial.

• A gift certificate for a makeover.

• A gift certificate for a trip to the beauty parlor.

• A gift certificate for a manicure or pedicure.

• Nightgown—one size fits all, opened down the front. These are available at Sears and all stores that carry fuller women's clothes. Even if the individual is not a fuller size, it is smart to have this kind of gown for the post-op period. Choose a pretty pastel color.

• A flower with a special card that tells her how special she is and how much she is loved.

• A gift certificate for a romantic dinner with the man she loves. If this gift is from a man, perhaps give just a card to let her know the date and time you plan to pick her up.

• A gift certificate for an overnight stay for two in a hotel with a Jacuzzi.

Valuable Information for the Husband or Significant Sweetie

The woman you love isn't going through this medical crisis alone. You feel the emotional pain and anxiety along with her. This is the time to show that you will stand behind her. A time to let her see that your love for her doesn't exist in the flesh that she is about to lose. Demonstrate your strength to her. She needs to rely on you to help her make personal decisions about treatment options. She also needs you to carry the load when it comes to her immediate recovery at home. The following books and suggestions may be helpful to you as you proceed down this path of transformation with your loved one.

Man to Man: When the Woman You Love Has Breast Cancer by Andy Murcia and Bob Stewart (St. Martin's Press, 1989)

This is a marvelous book written by Ann Jillian's husband and a close friend of theirs whose wife was also diagnosed with breast cancer, as Ann was. It is written for men. I wish I had known about this book during my diagnostic and treatment phases. You may need to place a special order for it from a bookstore, because I've found that many stores don't keep a ready supply in stock. Waldenbooks and B. Dalton can order it quickly (about 7 days).

Dr. Susan Love's Breast Book by Susan M. Love, M.D. (Perseus Press, 1995)

This book, referred to in more detail in Chapter 7, is worth the time it takes to read it. Although the drawings give you a sense of what to expect post-op, they are subtle. This book can also be listened to because it is also available on a CD.

Call her breast surgeon or family doctor for a private phone consultation.

A physician may be able to connect you with the mate of another woman who has weathered the storm of breast cancer in the recent past. A real sense of relief is created when talking to someone who has been there and made it through. If her physician is not helpful, the Reach to Recovery program might be.

Talk with clergy.

Sometimes we don't think to turn to those ready, willing, and able to help us. Prayer is a very powerful tool in the fight against cancer. Your church may have support group meetings or know of members who are also going through the trials of such a disease. Remember there is power in numbers.

Plan ahead. Make a schedule of things that must be done before, during, and after surgery.

Women are notorious for worrying, so spare her the additional stress of worrying about paying bills, finding sitters to watch the kids while she's in the hospital, and so on. Sit down and make a plan. If she insists, let her help you. Recruit family and friends to help with child care, pet care, fixing meals, etc. By planning ahead, you help her concentrate on getting well instead of on family crisis management. Everyone will sleep better if you plan.

Spend some time alone, just the two of you.

She needs to feel your strength and love. It is important to spend time talking about what she feels, and what she is most worried about. All too often we live in the fast lane and don't spend quality time together. If there was ever a time to rearrange priorities, this is it. Put her at the top of your list. Share your concerns with her. Most important, share your love.

Write down the questions you both have and take them to your doctor's appointments.

It's too easy to forget your questions once you are at the doctor's office and your adrenaline is pumping. A small notebook that will fit in your pocket makes a handy place to collect your questions.

Keep it with you all the time so it isn't forgotten on appointment days. Also record what your doctor says during the appointment, because when nerves are frazzled, memory can be affected.

Above all else, THINK POSITIVE!

If there is anyone who must remain optimistic, it is you. Breast cancer can be beaten! But surgery, radiation, and chemotherapy are only half the treatment. Your optimism and unrelenting love make up the other half. If you're feeling down, talk with someone you trust and can confide in. You are a very valuable key to her healing process.

DO's AND DON'TS FOR THE WOMAN ABOUT TO UNDERGO MASTECTOMY

DO take time to get all your questions answered by your physician. You deserve the answers; he or she owes you the time. Make a list of your questions and take the list with you when you have your next appointment.

DO purchase a large (one-size-fits-most/all) nightgown that buttons or snaps down the front. You will be much more comfortable in it than in your regular nightgowns when you come home from mastectomy surgery. These gowns have large armholes and are very flowing. There is room for you, your bandages, and your drainage tubes.

DO stock up on basic dressing supplies, such as a small box of 4x4 gauze pads and a roll of paper or adhesive tape. Though the hospital will send some home with you, it usually isn't enough.

DO let family and friends help. This is not the time to be a martyr. Let neighbors feed the dog (and the kids, for that matter) while you are in the hospital. Casseroles are always welcome. Let your sister vacuum for you, your husband do the dishes, and the kids clean up after themselves. Your recovery will be smoother and faster if you take the time to take care of yourself, not just those around you.

DO move your wristwatch from one wrist to the other if you are having a mastectomy on the side where you usually wear your watch. It is not advisable to wear anything constricting on the arm next to the affected area. This is because some or all of your lymph nodes will be removed. These glands carry fluid away from your upper extremities and help to ward off infection. Maintaining good circulation is further promoted by avoiding constricting objects such as tight-fitting rings and elastic sleeves.

DO share your thoughts and concerns with your spouse, other pertinent family members, and close friends. There is no reason to bear the burden alone. You'll feel better, and so will they.

DO get fitted for a wig before starting chemotherapy treatments (if this is part of your therapy). The fit will be better and, as a result, you will be happier with your appearance. Keep in mind that when your hair grows back, it will be healthier, fuller, and have more body than ever before. You'll never have another "bad hair day" again.

DO pamper yourself. Indulge in long, luxurious bubble baths, a trip to the sauna, a facial, or the purchase of that new perfume you've been wanting. I'm not suggesting that this is the time to spend your paycheck on frivolous things, but a $10 manicure can go a long way toward lifting your spirits on a day riddled with unpleasantness, such as receiving chemotherapy.

DO talk with your clergy and other religious people close to you to gain additional support during the trying times ahead. Placing your faith in God will help restore your mind to a sense of peace.

DON'T give all your bras away. You may be able to have them altered by sewing a pocket in them to hold your breast prosthesis. Check with stores that sell prostheses; they frequently know of women who alter bras as a full-time job. However, they don't usually advertise it.

DON'T give away all your swimsuits, either. It is very easy to have pockets sewn into most suits. It would be a shame to toss your favorite suit away without at least attempting to sew a pocket into it. Even if your suit is cut low, you can have what is called a "privacy panel" sewn in. This is a piece of cloth that matches the color/pattern of your suit and adds coverage to the upper portion of your swimsuit. These work very well.

DON'T assume you won't be attractive anymore. Trust me. Your bosom will get more attention after surgery than you ever remember it getting before. Just keep people guessing which is the live one and which is the Memorex. Only your surgeon, significant sweetie or husband, and hairdresser need to know for sure.

Appendix A

BREAST CANCER: MAKING THE RIGHT CHOICES FOR YOU

If you have just been diagnosed with breast cancer or have a strong suspicion that you might be, you're probably feeling overwhelmed, anxious, and powerless—all normal feelings when confronted with a disease that affects one in eight women in the United States. All too often, women travel blindly through the health-care system not knowing if they're in the best hands that they could be—and should be. For treatment of the common cold and other common disorders, it's fine to seek out care from local physicians who would normally provide you with primary care. When dealing with a life-threatening situation such as breast cancer, however, choosing the wrong doctor or the wrong breast center can be fatal. You must choose carefully and wisely. After all, we're talking about your life.

I am a breast cancer survivor. I am also a nurse. I've been where you are right now and know the anxiousness that you feel. For more than a decade, I was the director of quality of care and utilization management at Johns Hopkins Hospital, striving every day to measure and assess quality of care and work with the health-care professionals at the hospital to continuously improve the care we provide. I joined the team of the Johns Hopkins Breast Center to further accomplish this goal, but have chosen to channel all of my energies and expertise into the area of breast cancer. My goal is to make it easier for women like you who come behind me to also become one of the survivors like me.

There have been many women who came to the Johns Hopkins Breast Center who were seen by physicians elsewhere who didn't

provide them the ideal care and treatment they needed. This resulted in major medical problems for them long term—wrong
diagnosis, incomplete or inaccurate information, misleading information, and confusing information. As an institution committed to
patient care and teaching, we want to provide you some guidelines
as to how to go about choosing a physician and facility that's right
for you. We want you to know how to choose who will take good
care of you and give you your best opportunity to defeat this disease. The best answer isn't always the same for each person. We
want you to have the tools needed to make the very best choices for
you and your family in the battle against this disease.

Though a diagnosis of breast cancer is devastating to hear, it's
not something that requires emergency treatment. This is often a
misleading piece of information for women. They assume that
because they now have breast cancer that it must be treated immediately. Not true. Though delaying for a prolonged time period
(more than a couple of months) is not advisable, in most cases you
don't have to rush into making decisions. More importantly, if a
doctor tells you that you must have surgery immediately, take caution. If your cancer was diagnosed with either a mammogram or
because you or a physician felt a lump, the cancer has probably
been growing for five to eight years. It took a long time for a few
tiny cells to mature enough to become a tumor which could be seen
on an X-ray or felt. So you don't have to have surgery right away.
You don't have to make hurried decisions without adequate information about your treatment options and about what's really best
for you. You have time to gather information. You have time to
seek out the best doctors and facilities to take care of you.

At a time when you feel powerless having heard the verdict of
breast cancer, it's important to seek out constructive ways to
empower yourself once again and gain some control over your life
and the situation placed before you. The breast cancer specialists of
the Johns Hopkins Breast Center are strong believers in the value
of providing women with information about their disease and its
treatment options. An informed patient is a patient who will do well

psychologically. An informed patient is someone who can participate in the decision-making about her care and feel confident in the
choices made. An informed patient knows what to expect along
each step of the way from point of diagnosis through to completion
of treatment and beyond so that she's actually a member of her own
health-care team. She should be an equal partner with the breast
cancer specialists who have her best interests in mind—survival,
good quality of life, and confidence in the choices made about her
health and well-being.

We've spoken to patients who have been to other physicians
elsewhere who made them feel pressured to proceed quickly with
treatment before they'd had time to think things through and really participate in the decision-making about what was best for them.
If you're confronted with a doctor who's pressuring you to have
surgery right away or who is not informing you about what all your
options are, you need to seek care elsewhere. In the same light,
you'll also need to seek care elsewhere if you're being told by a
doctor information that sounds too good to be true compared to
opinions you have gotten elsewhere. For example, if you've been
told that you probably have a large tumor and/or positive lymph
nodes based on physical exam, biopsy results, and mammography
which would definitely require chemotherapy as part of your treatment, don't be fooled by a doctor who tells you "if you have your
treatment here, you won't need chemotherapy." It simply isn't true
and isn't logical. Though getting good news like this from another
physician can at first sound great, if you've done your homework
and studied up on your clinical situation, you would know that this
doesn't sound right. Don't be fooled by such an opinion. Get a third
opinion if you need it. You're far better off with a breast cancer
specialist who tells you frankly and honestly what your situation is
than to have someone paint a rosy picture which in the end isn't so
rosy.

The decisions you make can and will affect the rest of your life.
That's why it's so important that you empower yourself with information so that you can determine for yourself if you're in good

hands. It doesn't mean that you have to have a medical degree, either. It does mean that you need to take some time and read about breast cancer, the various treatments that are available to treat this disease, and how to best determine what will be the right choices for your situation. You also have time to gather information through reading literature. Many sources are helpful in explaining in layman's terms what the nature of this disease is all about, what types of surgery are done, and what types of adjuvant therapy (chemotherapy and radiation therapy) are available to eradicate this disease and have you become a long-term survivor.

So how do I start? You start by taking a deep breath, sitting down, talking to family and friends who can offer you emotional support, and tackling this new crisis one step at a time. Below is a guide to help you become an empowered, informed woman who will have the knowledge and resources needed to make decisions confidently about your breast cancer treatment.

Choosing a doctor. Once you've been told that you do have breast cancer or might have breast cancer, you'll be referred to a surgeon. There are many doctors who perform breast cancer surgery, but not that many who are truly breast surgeons. Breast surgery, whether it be in the form of a lumpectomy or mastectomy, has historically been thought to be a "simple" surgical procedure to do. Well, if it's your breast, it might not sound so simple. There are many general surgeons who perform breast cancer surgery. They might do one case a year or perhaps as many as twenty. You want to go and be seen by a surgeon who IS a breast surgeon ...who has chosen this to be his or her surgical specialty and who does a lot of breast surgeries every year. These are physicians with the surgical experience you're seeking. They've chosen this as their field of specialty and will probably be more up-to-date on the latest surgical techniques. High-volume surgeons tend to have better results and are more attuned to subtle differences in individual cases. Seek out a physician who does fifty or more breast cancer operations a year. (For example, in Maryland during 1996, there were 287 surgeons who performed only one inpatient breast cancer surgery.

There were an additional ninety-four physicians who only did two such operations. Of all the women having breast cancer surgery in Maryland during this period, only 8.6 percent of them were treated by a surgeon who had done more than fifty breast surgical procedures that year. Additionally, of the 647 surgeons who did inpatient breast cancer surgery, only 1.5 percent of them had done more than thirty inpatient operations in 1996.) You can find out this kind of information from several sources: Call the hospital where the doctor is in practice and ask for information about case volume. The physician's office should be more than willing to provide this type of information to you. Call your state board of quality assurance and ask for information on file about the physician you're considering. They will also have information about any malpractice cases he/she has had and other quality-of-care complaints that have been filed against him/her. This information isn't published data but is available by making a simple call. (Keep in mind, however, that physicians who treat large numbers of women with breast cancer may have some information on file whereas a physician who treats only a handful of patients in a year may have nothing on file.)

You also want to know about the credentialing of the physicians you choose; this includes your breast surgeon, medical oncologist, radiation oncologist, radiologist, and others involved in your care. Your wisest choice is to choose a physician board-certified by The American Board of Surgery as your breast surgeon. He or she has to be trained in recognized, approved training programs and pass rigorous exams after training. The American Board of Medical Specialists can be reached by calling (847) 491-9091 or by going to their website: www.aabms.org/abms/. They can provide you with information regarding who in your region meets these criteria. Surgeons of this specialty also frequently are members of the American College of Surgeons. This distinction comes only after having become board certified and practicing in a community for more than three years. These surgeons are considered by their peers to be above-average in the care of surgical patients.

Finally, most true breast surgeons are also members of The

Society of Surgical Oncology. This society only accepts as members those with substantially greater training and/or experience in the management of cancer. Most of the latest developments in the surgical management of breast cancer patients are presented at annual educational meetings of this society. The standards for the surgical care of breast cancer patients are developed by the American College of Surgeons and The Society of Surgical Oncology jointly.

Not all breast surgeons do breast cancer surgeries 100 percent of the time. But consider this—some full-time breast surgeons do surgery on only twenty-five to thirty new cancer patients each year, but others who do only 75 percent breast surgery treat more than 200 new cases a year!

The same criteria apply for each other specialty physician who will be providing your care. They should be board certified for their specialty with a subspecialty in breast cancer. There are lots of physicians, for example, who are medical oncologists and provide treatment to cancer patients. You want to receive your care, however, from someone whose specialty or major interest is breast cancer.

Physician attitude. Seek out someone who's going to be very frank and honest with you. This is not the time to have a sugared version of what your situation is. You need the facts and you want them presented to you candidly. This can be emotionally difficult for some physicians, so you never really end up with the whole, unvarnished truth. Seek out a physician who's willing to spend time with you and answer all your questions. No physician knows all—they should be willing to discuss the uncertainties in treatment and results. Beware of the omniscient doctor. That person may not be able to recognize their shortcomings or see alternatives in treatment that may not be the usual local treatment policy.

Seek a physician who wants to help educate you about this disease and your treatment options—not someone who wants to make the decisions for you. Remember, you need to be part of your own treatment team. That is important. It can be tempting to just have the doctor tell you what to do, but that really isn't in your best interest. There are critical choices that you must make which need to be your decision alone. One example is whether to have mastectomy or breast conservation surgery (lumpectomy with lymph node removal). Depending on your clinical condition and the size of the tumor, along with some other factors, it may very well be that from a survival perspective, you will be given the choice of having one type of surgery or the other, both having equal outcomes regarding your survival rate. This is a decision that should be left for you to decide based on many factors, including your emotional well-being and the feelings you have about your self-image. You, not the doctor, will face the consequences of these decisions for the rest of your life. Make sure these decisions and treatments have your seal of approval.

Talk with other survivors. Getting information from other women who are breast cancer survivors can be very valuable. Also, take comfort in knowing that there are many of us who HAVE survived this disease (there are 1.3 million breast cancer survivors in the U.S. today). These women can give you candid information about their own experiences with physicians who provided them care and treatment when they were diagnosed. It's best to talk with someone who has been treated fairly recently, though, because treatment modalities change. For example, if you spoke to someone who had a mastectomy seven years ago, she'd tell you that she spent several days in the hospital and suffered with nausea and vomiting and a lot of pain. Physicians who have chosen to continuously improve care for women battling breast cancer will make changes in their surgical care to prevent the side effects that women in the past had to overcome. There are various types of surgical treatments for breast cancer, too, and you'll find that the experiences women share with you, based on the type of surgery they had, also will vary. The results also vary dramatically between hospitals and individual doctors. Don't expect the good results from one hospital to translate into similar results at others.

For example, women having mastectomies or lumpectomies

with lymph node removal and not having reconstruction at the same time should describe an experience free of severe pain and absence of nausea and vomiting. However, the reported rates of nausea and vomiting in most hospitals in the country exceed 85 percent. Several years ago, we at Johns Hopkins pioneered improvements in anesthesia management and other peri-operative surgical care so that the majority of our women patients can awaken from this type of surgery and feel relatively normal from a physical perspective. I know our own experience at Hopkins since 1995 has been that women undergoing one of these two procedures without reconstruction feel well enough to go home the same day.

The emotional aspects of this disease and its treatment cannot be underplayed. We want patients to focus on addressing their emotional needs as a priority and not have to worry about feeling ill from surgery. If you find that previous patients you speak to are describing unpleasant experiences from their surgical event, you might want to get more information before selecting the same doctor that they chose. There will be other important services to ask former patients about, too, which will be described in more detail below (such as the ease of reaching a health-care professional if you need to after you go home.)

Multi-disciplinary care. Lots of facilities boast that they offer this. What does it really mean, though? Multi-disciplinary means that you're being seen and cared for by a team of breast cancer specialists with expertise in breast surgery, medical oncology, radiation oncology, plastic surgery, cytopathology, and mammography with diagnostic imaging. Some hospitals or breast centers have such a team. This team may be, however, the only team, meaning that they only have one medical oncologist or one breast surgeon. Ideally, you want to go to a place where there are several physicians of each specialty and where your specific case will be discussed and reviewed by the specific team caring for you, as well as by the other physicians there who can offer second opinions on an ongoing basis. In most cases, the types of facilities that offer this level of faculty staffing are at larger teaching hospitals. It's important to have this type of specialized care and expertise, however. Each step of your care is too important to delegate to a single individual—only through open review and debate of each step in the treatment process can the ideal treatment and management be certain.

Skill, knowledge, and technology. The effective treatment of your breast cancer is critical for you. You deserve to receive your care in the most up-to-date facility where the latest and newest technology for diagnosing and treating breast cancer is available. The physicians and nurses who care for you should be specialized in the diagnosis and treatment of breast cancer. There are always new research and innovative treatments being developed for this disease. Having your care at a facility that can offer state-of-the-art diagnostic evaluation and treatment should be your priority. Being able to have access to the latest treatment modalities, including clinical trials for treatment of breast cancer, will be valuable for you. Don't settle for a program that's limited in what it can provide to you.

For example, facilities that offer state-of-the-art biopsies in the form of "percutaneous biopsies" are ideal. Percutaneous biopsies mean that you can be biopsied in mammography by a radiologist who has been specially trained. The physician can remove tissue for further examination by a pathologist without having to put you to sleep. Doing the procedure this way is less painful and allows most women to do it on their lunch hour and get the results within twenty-four hours. If the facility you've chosen doesn't have such equipment or professional expertise, you expose yourself to having procedures done the old-fashioned way, which may limit some of your future treatment options.

Features of a breast center. You'll note that I chose to say "breast center." I guess that's my own bias. I believe that you have a better opportunity of having a truly integrated and comprehensive program for diagnosing and treating breast cancer if the facility has chosen to invest in developing a center for breast health and the treatment of breast cancer. Tagging the word "center" onto a title, though, doesn't mean it is one. There are certain features of a breast center that you should expect to be offered as part of their program if they are, in fact, truly a comprehensive breast center. I've listed some of them below for you.

Easy access. If you've been advised to see a surgeon due to an abnormal mammogram or lump discovered on examination, you'll want an appointment as soon as possible. Until you're seen by a surgeon and answers are known about your clinical situation, your anxiety and stress level will remain high. Most breasts centers, in acknowledgment of this, will (and should) schedule you for an appointment within forty-eight hours of your call or a doctor's referral. Fear of the unknown is the worst fear of all. Even if the news you receive is bad, you can take comfort in knowing that now you can begin working with the doctors to plan what will be the best treatment choices for you.

Patient empowerment. It's important that you be given the knowledge you need to enable you to actively participate in decisions about your care and treatment. Some physicians are reluctant to empower women in this way. It's a patient's right and should be a key factor in deciding where you want to receive your treatment.

Patient education. Not only do you need to be educated about breast cancer, the treatment options, and what to expect each step along the way, but so do important members of your family. This requires an investment of time and resources by the health-care professionals taking care of you. You want to receive and be educated about your treatment plans as thoroughly as possible. You need to have easy access to someone in the breast center that you can ask questions of and feel confident in the responses as well as comfortable asking the questions. By doing so, you'll come to understand what's happening to your body and what needs to be done for you to get well again. Your family members who love you and need to support you benefit from this education, too, because they're worried about you. They need to understand what's happening so they can devote their time and energy to emotionally supporting you.

Multi-disciplinary case conferences. A key advantage to having a multi-disciplinary team approach is the special expertise each health-care professional offers to each patient's unique situation. Centers that routinely hold case conferences to discuss in detail a patient's clinical condition, diagnostic findings, and recommendations for optimal treatment are beneficial to the patient's overall well-being and clinical outcome. This is a way to help ensure that the patient is being given individualized attention and care by utilizing maximum breast cancer knowledge, experience, and expertise by the breast center team.

Special mammography services.

Appointments right away. If a woman is being referred by her family doctor or gynecologist for evaluation of a suspicious lump, she wants to know right away if it's cancer. For that matter, if she finds the lump herself, she doesn't want there to be any delay in getting the answers about her situation. Mammography facilities should offer appointments for such patients immediately. Ideally, the patient would be seen the same day, or at the latest, the following day. Oftentimes, radiologists are not readily available to read the films and talk with the patient about what the mammogram showed. You want to go to a facility that has radiologists available to read the films while you're there and most importantly, tell you what they show. Be sure to call and ask whether they offer this type of clinical service. It's one additional way to reduce your anxiety and speed the process along for you to get answers and proceed with treatment if it's determined to be cancer.

Percutaneous biopsy—mammotome, ABBI, core biopsy, and fine needle biopsies. These are four types of biopsy procedures that can now be done in mammography if the facility has the technology and medical expertise. This method of doing breast biopsies enables the patient to have a sample of tissue removed without having an open biopsy requiring an incision. Having the biopsy done this way requires special equipment and devices that not all mammography facilities currently have. It also requires special credentialing for the radiologist doing this type of procedure.

Learning about these programs and services is an additional way to judge how up-to-date the facility that you're considering is.

Inform the patient and referring physician of the findings right away. Once you've had a biopsy, you'll want to know the results as soon as possible. Check to see what the turnaround time is for the pathology results. Many facilities can tell you or your doctor the results of a biopsy within twenty-four hours. The sooner you know what you're dealing with, the sooner you can begin to make plans about the best treatment options for you to pursue.

Clinical trials. Having available to you as many treatment options as possible is important. Hospitals which participate in clinical trials can usually offer more innovative treatment options. In some cases, these clinical trials are very new and the medical field is still learning about all of their benefits and value. If you're asked to participate in such a trial, you'll be paving the way to the development of innovative research that will make an important impact on other women diagnosed with breast cancer in the future. You're also being closely monitored throughout your treatment process so that data can be collected about your experience with the chemotherapy agents you've been given. You might also be asked to participate in a study that has already proven to be very beneficial for treating breast cancer and now different dosages are being tested to determine the optimal dosage and frequency for you and other patients treated in the future. These new discoveries not only benefit you today but also will make a big difference in how many lives we save in the future.

State-of-the-art breast cancer surgery with minimal pain and nausea-free. Most surgeons would say that doing a mastectomy or lumpectomy isn't technically complicated surgery to perform. That doesn't mean, however, than any general surgeon does the procedure well. It's very important to have breast cancer surgery done by a surgeon who has chosen breast cancer surgery to be his or her surgical specialty and who does a large volume of breast surgeries on an annual basis. Historically, it was common for women to experience nausea, vomiting, and postoperative pain following lumpectomy or mastectomy surgery, even those not having reconstruction done at the same time. There are breast centers that have resolved this chronic problem and now are able to perform this type of surgery with minimal discomfort and without the gastrointestinal side effects oftentimes accompanying general anesthesia. It's important to ask questions related to this. The doctors who you're considering should have quality-of-care data that describes their nausea/vomiting rate, pain management, average length of time in the hospital for surgery with and without reconstruction, complications that occur during or after surgery, and satisfaction data from prior patients' experience—all important information when choosing who you want to have take care of you. At Hopkins, for women who have breast cancer surgery without reconstruction, the majority of patients feel so physically well after surgery that they choose to go home that same day. They're visited by a home health-care nurse that evening and the next morning and are in constant contact with the nurse practitioner in their breast center for updates. What's nice about the option to go home is that it's the woman's choice. She is pain-free and nausea-free and able to concentrate on her emotional well-being, which should be her primary focus postoperatively.

Radiation oncology. Patients who undergo lumpectomy surgery for treatment of their breast cancer almost always receive this form of adjuvant therapy afterward. Most hospitals offer radiation oncology services. If the type of treatment advised for you includes radiation therapy, you'll want to ask questions about the radiation oncology physician's experience with treating breast cancer patients. Again, it's valuable to go to a facility that has extensive experience with treating this specific type of cancer. They should also have a physicist on staff who assists with this type of treatment to help ensure that the radiation is done in the precise location where the treatment is needed. As is the case with all of your treatment, you as a patient should be given the opportunity to participate in the decision-making about this type of treatment option. The physicians and nurses should be forthcoming with information about how this treatment is done, the risks and benefits of it, and precisely how it will be administered to you.

Plastic surgery offering the latest techniques.
   Free-flap reconstructive surgery. Most hospitals and breast centers have plastic surgeons who can perform flap reconstruction by taking tissues from other parts of your body (usually the tummy area) and creating from it a new breast. This, in the past, required the surgeon to maintain all of the vascular system (blood flow) attached during the procedure. There are new techniques now being used which enable the surgeon to transplant this tissue, cutting the vessels free. By using intricate microvascular surgery, the plastic surgeon is then able to reconstruct the arteries and veins in their new location. The result for the patient is less pain after surgery. There are only a few facilities, however, who have a surgeon with expertise in this type of procedure. If you're considering having this type of reconstruction done, you may want to ask about this new method. Again, it's also important that the plastic surgeon you choose be someone who has done a large volume of flap- and free-flap reconstructive breast surgeries. Experience is a valuable asset when you want the very best cosmetic results that can be achieved.
   Skin-sparing mastectomy. This is also a fairly new form of surgery, which was developed at Hopkins and other major cancer centers. The affected breast is hollowed out and then the tissue from the abdominal area is used to fill the opening and create a new breast. There are a few facilities that have the surgical expertise to perform this state-of-the-art breast cancer surgery/reconstruction combination. Talk with your surgeon about it and discuss the pros and cons of taking this approach. Again, the cosmetic appearance is amazing. When you see photographs of reconstructed breasts, you'll be impressed with this surgical cosmetic effect. Often, the patient doesn't look like she's had a mastectomy procedure done.
   Medical oncology. Most, but not all, patents diagnosed with breast cancer need some form of chemotherapy as part of their treatment. Again, most hospitals offer such clinical services. You

want to make sure that the medical oncologist overseeing your treatment is specialized in the treatment of breast cancer. A medical oncologist may treat a wide variety of patients with various forms of cancer. You want to be cared for by someone who has chosen to specialize in breast cancer treatment—someone who treats lots of women with this disease and has a track record for good outcomes. Ask the doctor about how many patients he or she treats in a given year for breast cancer and ask about the patients' experience with complications from the treatment. You want to have a board-certified medical oncologist who is readily accessible in the event that you need to talk with him or her urgently while going through treatment. Ask questions about the doctor's procedure for addressing emergency calls as well as what type of monitoring will be done while you are undergoing this type of adjuvant therapy. Ask about the survival statistics for breast cancer patients treated at the facility you're considering, too.

All cancer patients' data is entered into a national database giving cancer specialists the ability to compare various treatment modalities and clinical outcomes. Hospitals who treat large volumes of cancer patients also study their own data and compare it to national statistics. You want to be in the hands of a team of professionals who have a history of good outcomes. Whenever possible, seek care at a facility which can demonstrate that their survival rate is better than the national average. (For example, at Hopkins, for women who are premenopausal and have positive lymph notes, the survival rate is 10 percent higher than the national average.) You will have a higher sense of confidence and security being treated in a place that has these types of results.

Autologous Bone Marrow Transplant (ABMT). This is a very specialized procedure which is done when very aggressive treatment is recommended. The patient has her healthy bone marrow harvested and stored away for safekeeping. She then receives high doses of chemotherapy, which, as a side effect, destroys her remaining marrow. Afterward, her healthy bone marrow is returned to her. If a bone marrow transplant is advised for your type of breast cancer treatment, you'll want to select where you go care-fully. Your insurance carrier may have a special arrangement with specific hospitals in your area or farther away since this type of treatment isn't done at very many places. If given the option, you want to be able to have all of your care at one facility where conti-nuity of care can be provided smoothly. If you do need this type of treatment, go to a facility that has experience with doing large vol-umes of bone marrow transplants specifically for the treatment of breast cancer. The more experienced the doctors and nurses are with this type of treatment, the better your personal care and clini-cal outcomes will probably be. As a new state-of-the-art approach for ABMT, a few, but very few, facilities are doing the procedure in the way that can reduce the amount of time the patient needs to spend hospitalized, which is usually several weeks. For example, Hopkins has a program called "IPOP" which stands for "inpa-tient/outpatient" bone marrow transplant. Breast cancer patients are kept in the acute hospital bed for as brief a time as is absolutely needed and receive a large majority of their treatment and intensive monitoring in an outpatient setting located at the hospital. This enables the patient to spend more time with family while receiving this life-saving treatment to help eradicate her breast cancer.

Genetic counseling. This is a special program for women who have a family history of breast cancer or have other factors that make them higher risk for developing this disease. Counseling and genetic testing require specialists who not only are experts in this field but also have excellent communication skills. The choice to have counseling and especially to decide to proceed with genetic testing is one to be taken seriously and with some caution. Though it can sound simple to be tested, there are many things to consider before making such a choice. Physicians and nurses who have cho-sen to specialize in this field have expertise with helping women make these choices. Currently, only a few facilities offer this type of program; it's a growing field, however. If this is an area of inter-est to you or your family, you want to go to a facility that has many years of experience with genetic counseling and testing for breast cancer. Ask how long their program has existed and how many patients have been counseled and tested during that time. This will give you some idea as to their experience with this specialized type of service.

High-risk assessment for breast cancer. Being evaluated for your risk of developing breast cancer or a family member getting this disease may be important for you. There are health-care professionals who specialize in this type of screening and evaluation. Ask the breast center where you're contemplating going for your care if they offer this service, who performs the service, and how many patients they screen a year. The program should be conducted by a doctor or a nurse practitioner who specializes in breast health screening programs.

Pathology services. Patients don't always think about this particular service, but it's a very important one. The pathologist who looks at your tissue specimen determines what type of breast cancer you have, how fast it's growing, whether it has spread to your lymph nodes, and provides other important pieces of clinical information to your breast surgeon, medical oncologist, and radiation oncologist. Accuracy and completeness are critical. It's difficult for a layperson to assess whether the pathology services being provided at a hospital are of good quality or not. One source for this information is the Joint Commission on Accreditation of Healthcare Organizations (JCAHO). They inspect hospitals on a tri-annual basis and write up reports on their findings. Included in their inspection are their findings for the pathology department. Though they don't actually look at slides and determine if they were accurately interpreted, they do look at the processes used by pathology to determine how effectively they work. They also review the credential files of the pathologists and other faculty at the facility. You can see the latest results of the hospital's inspection by going to the JCAHO website at www.jcaho.org or calling (630) 792-5800 and requesting a copy of the report. This information became publicly accessible in 1997. There are some pathology departments who have made errors in reading the results of a breast tissue specimen. The worst case is when a specimen is read as benign tissue when in fact it contains cancer cells. You may wish to consider obtaining a second opinion about the pathology results by taking your pathology slides to a second facility that has extensive experience in diagnosing and treating breast cancer. The pathologist should be considered one of the members of the breast center team and actively participate in the case conferences referenced earlier in this book. The information they provide serves as the road map for determining the treatment plan options best for your specific situation. Ask if the pathologist attends these conferences and what role he or she plays in the actual case discussion.

Patient satisfaction surveys. There are a few breast centers who perform patient satisfaction surveys, but all should. It's important to learn from patients how satisfied they were with their care and how the center can improve specific services and programs offered to make care even better than before. Conducting surveys is time- and resource-intensive. Centers who have chosen to survey their patients are sending an important message—that the health-care professionals there care about their patients' opinions and want to hear from them. When asking a breast center whether they conduct surveys or not, also ask what they do with the results they obtain. It's one thing to collect the data; it's another to do something constructive with it. Health-care professionals need to take their patients' opinions seriously. All too often, a patient may complain about a specific service or aspect of care she received and her words are not taken to heart. Seek out a place where the philosophy of the center is to use the results of their patient satisfaction surveys to determine what initiatives the center will work on to improve patient care. Go to a facility that considers the patients' opinions the most valuable—even more valuable than the health-care professionals taking care of the patient. (A doctor may think it's acceptable for a patient to wait two weeks for an appointment when she has found a lump in her breast; the patient feels, however, that she should be able to get an appointment that same week. The patient is right!) Breast centers that truly have the patients' best interests in mind will demonstrate this philosophy by conducting surveys and acting on the results in real time.

Continuity of care. As more and more health-care services are converted from an inpatient setting to an outpatient setting, the need to ensure effective and efficient continuity of care heightens. Ask the facility how they go about keeping your primary-care doctor or referring physician aware of your condition and treatment status. Check to see how they manage to keep track of how you're doing after you go home following surgery or chemotherapy treatments. Ask who is responsible for coordinating your care. You need to have confidence that you're being watched over even when you're not physically in the hospital. Some facilities have nurse practitioners that stay in touch with their patients via telephone once patients are home. Some facilities offer home-health nursing care after surgical treatment is done. The team of professionals taking care of you also needs to stay in close contact with one another—that's why they're a team. Ask them how they communicate with one another and keep each other informed about your progress and needs. You want to be cared for by a team who stays well-connected with you and with one another, including your referring physician or doctor who functions as your family doctor. Feeling confidant that you're receiving good continuity of care provides wonderful peace of mind to you and your family.

Urgent-care needs services. When an urgent problem arises (such as a sickness that won't subside following a treatment), you need to have ready access to a professional who can take care of this situation promptly. Ask what the breast center's procedures are for handling such emergencies. Also ask how often patients in the past have needed to utilize this special service. A breast center should have available for its patients a professional health-care provider twenty-four hours a day, seven days a week to handle emergencies. In addition to this, the patients should be well-informed about how to access this urgent-care service and know that they can confidently rely on it. You shouldn't have to go to an emergency room to have your urgent-care needs attended. If their patient education program is thorough and well-done, you and your family will know how to take care of most crises and head them off at the pass. (For example, taking an anti-nausea drug at a designated time to prevent vomiting later on.) There are unforeseen circumstances, however, that do arise and warrant prompt intervention by a doctor or nurse. Knowing and understanding how urgent-care needs are handled is important. Though you may never need to use it, you want to know that such a program is in place and works well.

Long-term follow-up. Some doctors take care of your breast cancer and when treatment is done, send you back to your referring physician. Their involvement with you ends when treatment ends. From a continuity of care perspective, as well as peace of mind, it's better to be cared for by professionals who will continue to see you for the rest of your life. Though we hope that your breast cancer does not recur, there is a possibility that it might. Having the same health-care team who treated you from the start continue to follow you at designated intervals to ensure that you remain well and healthy is a smart thing. Ask the center what its protocol is for following patients after their treatment is completed. You have been through a life-threatening experience and need to continue to be seen, screened, and evaluated by the people who are intimately familiar with your history and the treatment that was done.

Psychological support for you and your family. Being diagnosed with breast cancer is devastating. Though some people don't openly express how they feel, it's impossible not to be upset when told you have breast cancer. Those who love you are distressed, too. Having ready access to professionals who can offer guidance, support, and help you and your family develop coping skills will make your breast cancer treatment go more smoothly for everyone. Ask the facility if it offers such services. You want to talk with professionals who have extensive experience with breast cancer patients and their families, who are familiar with the treatment you'll be receiving and know the doctors and nurses involved in your care. This provides for a better-integrated approach to getting you well again physically and emotionally. A few facilities offer private counseling and psychotherapy. Most also have breast cancer support groups who generally meet monthly and are facilitated by a social worker or nurse. Some facilities also offer special support programs for family members, including husbands and young children.

Survivor support. When confronted with a diagnosis of breast cancer, your initial thought may be that you're alone in this battle. Feel assured you are not. There are 1.3 million women who are breast cancer survivors living in the Unites States today. Many breast centers arrange for breast cancer survivors to talk with women who are newly diagnosed with this disease. The American Cancer Society offers, as a free service, a program called "Reach to Recovery." This program matches newly diagnosed women with women who are of the same or similar culture, ethnicity, and clinical condition (for example matching a forty-something-year-old with stage II breast cancer who's having a mastectomy and chemotherapy with a woman who's also in her forties and had the same treatment modality in the past and has completed her treatment at least a year ago). This program is designed to help address the emotional needs you'll be having. There's great benefit in talking to someone who has been through what you're about to go through. Some breast centers have taken this program a step further and arrange for their own breast cancer survivor volunteers to also contact the patient. These survivor volunteers are very familiar with your situation because they've received their care from the same team of professionals you're receiving care from now. (Hopkins offers such a program. Though it's fairly new, it has already proven to be very beneficial for our patients and their families.) Different facilities and doctors have sometimes-different ways of doing certain types of treatments. Having a survivor who's familiar with the treatment program you're going to receive makes it easier to talk with and gain insight from her. This survivor volunteer becomes an extension of your breast cancer health-care team. Ask the facility you're considering if they offer such a program and how it's organized. There are some facilities that discourage having newly diagnosed patients talk with women who have been previously diagnosed and treated. The belief, in such situations, is that the survivor may in some way negatively influence the patient in her decision-making process. Health-care professionals need to recognize the value of new patients talking with patients who have had similar treatment in the past and allow them time to exchange information. It's a patient's right to gain as much insight and understanding about her disease and its treatment as she can. This is one additional method to accomplish this goal...and an additional way for you to evaluate the breast center you're considering.

Lymphedema prevention and management. A few patients, after having lymph nodes removed as part of their breast cancer surgery, develop lymphedema. This results in problems with swelling of their arm and hand on the side where their surgery was done. One way to prevent this from occurring is to be proactive in its management. Check to see if the breast center you're considering offers a "lymphedema prevention and management program." Such centers will have a certified occupational therapist or physical therapist become certified and credentialed in lymphedema management. The therapist will see the patient prior to her surgery and teach her special exercises to do to help prevent the chance of developing lymphedema. She also will help in managing the problem should it occur anyway. A few breast centers also offer special programs designed to prevent it and manage it—it's a sign of the comprehensiveness of their services.

Rehabilitation medicine. Having breast cancer surgery, whether it be a mastectomy or lumpectomy with lymph node removal, results in temporary difficulty with range of motion to your affected arm. It's smart to learn in advance of surgery the best exercises to prevent range-of-motion problems from occurring. Some breast centers offer, as part of their preoperative management and preparation, a program specifically for this. It's usually conducted by the Rehabilitation and Physical Medicine Department, which works in a coordinated manner with the breast center staff. Patients are trained in appropriate exercises to do by a physical therapist or occupational therapist. Patients who are experiencing problems with gaining their full range of motion back after their surgery are also seen by the same therapist. The therapist works with the patient to restore her physical abilities to what they were before. Most patients don't need assistance after surgery if they've been trained well and follow the prescribed exercise program shown to them. It's good to know that such programs exist, though, should you be in need of these special services.

Continued education programs and seminars. When your treatment is over, you'll still want to stay on top of the latest treatment programs and research discoveries being made about breast cancer. Your continued good health may depend on it. Most women thirst for information and want to learn as much as they can—it may make a difference for their own health or for someone in their family who they care about. Check to see what type of continued educational programs the facility offers related to breast cancer. Examples of seminars that might be offered include: hormone replacement therapy after breast cancer treatment; breast cancer gene research findings; the latest in breast reconstruction; and coping with fear of recurrence of breast cancer. Though your treatment may be over, the disease and its long-term effects may continue. You'll want to stay informed and updated at routine intervals.

Other cancer screening programs for you and your family. Breast cancer, though it may be happening to you, affects your entire family. Usually, a diagnosis of breast cancer is a surprise. This is the time to check out your health in general and that of your family to make sure that there are no other surprises. Men, at a minimum, should be checked for colon cancer and prostate cancer. Women need to also be checked for colon cancer and uterine cancer. Take this opportunity to commit to yourself and to your family to be properly screened for these types of cancers and others that may apply due to family history or lifestyle. See what types of cancer screening programs are offered at the facility where you plan to receive your care. Your family will thank you and you will thank yourself for having had the screening done. The outcome for everyone will be a healthier future.

Image recovery. There are side effects, physical ones and psychological ones, that can take a toll on us as women when we're treated for breast cancer. Some of us may lose a breast; others may lose our hair; many will lose both. These are symbols of femininity for many and are devastating to experience. Being prepared for these losses is a good way to adjust and cope. Some facilities offer on-site or have an affiliation with an "image recovery" service. These places are sometimes referred to as mastectomy supply shops, wig shops, or called by some other name. Their purpose is to help restore (with a breast prosthesis) or temporarily replace (with a wig) that which is lost from your self-image. If you anticipate needing a breast prosthesis, be sure to be fitted by someone who is a certified fitter. This individual would have taken a special course to learn how to properly fit a woman for a breast prosthesis. An improper fit can result in poor body alignment, back pain, and lack of confidence in one's appearance. Check to see what the facility has to offer and go and visit it if possible. Many of them also offer special classes in make-up and hairstyling as additional ways to improve our self-image and help us to feel good about our appearance. Remember, you need to not just physically heal but also to emotionally heal. Your treatments will go smoother if you can feel confident in the way you look during and after therapy.

Conclusion. I've tried to provide you some guidance and direction as to how to choose a breast center worthy of taking care of you. You are important...your care is important...it shouldn't be done just anywhere. After all, this is a life-altering experience, and depending on the accuracy of your diagnosis and effectiveness of your treatment, a life-saving experience. I want you to choose well. If you have questions or wish to discuss this one-on-one with me, you're welcome to reach me at the Johns Hopkins Breast Center. Remember, I am a breast cancer survivor. My mission is for there to be a lot more fellow survivors. Good luck to you, and I wish you well as you embark on your road of transformation from victim to breast cancer survivor.

Appendix B

ADDITIONAL RESOURCES YOU MAY FIND BENEFICIAL

Books:

Dr. Susan Love's Breast Book
By Susan Love, M.D. (Perseus, 1995).

This book is written in layman's terms and provides information about what breast cancer is and the various treatments that may be needed. There are subtle drawings of what surgical treatments look like as well as what various cell structures look like. The book is very good but can be overwhelming to read because it contains so much information. Choose the parts that are of most interest to your and your situation. The book is divided into chapters, which makes it easy to focus on specific areas of interest and concern. The book is available in most bookstores or can be ordered through amazon.com.

Will I Get Breast Cancer? Questions and Answers for Teenage Girls
By Carole G. Vogel (Julian Messner, 1995).

This is an exceptional book for teenagers who have a family history of breast cancer. Once a woman has breast cancer, she worries about the risks posed to her daughters as well. This book answers basic questions clearly and simply for teenage girls and their moms. It also provides information on what steps a young girl can take to improve her odds of not getting breast cancer by practicing good health prevention programs (which are described in detail.) It also takes some of the mystery out of the disease by explaining what breast cancer is, how it occurs and how it's treated. Most importantly, it provides hope for future generations. This book usually has to be ordered at a local bookstore.

Man to Man: When the Woman You Love Has Breast Cancer
By Andy Murcia and Bob Stewart (St. Martin's Press, 1989).
This book was written by Ann Jillian's husband and a close friend of theirs whose wife was diagnosed with breast cancer along with Ann. It's written for men and provides a candid description of the emotional roller-coaster that men experience when the woman they love is diagnosed with this disease. Men are not usually very good about expressing their emotions. This book is good for women to read so they can begin to understand what concerns their spouse/boyfriend may be experiencing. It's valuable for men to read so they can understand that the feelings they're having aren't exclusive to themselves but are common feelings men have. Men worry a lot...much more than they're usually able to overtly express. This book may give both of you insight into this and help open the doors of communication for yourselves, too. This book usually needs to be ordered from a local chain bookstore and is available in just a few days.

Courage & Cancer
By Marilyn R. Moody (Rhache Publishers, 1996).
This is a breast cancer diary, consisting of a series of letters the author wrote to her best friend. Although she lived across the country from the author, her friend was her primary support system from the time she was initially diagnosed to the completion of her treatment. It's very good—you experience their emotions with them, and share their triumph in the end. This book can be special ordered through amazon.com.

Information Sources:

**The Cancer Information Service of
the National Cancer Institute
(800) 4-CANCER
http://rex.nci.nih.gov**
This organization provides information about all types of cancer,

including excellent information about breast cancer: what it is, how it's treated, and where various treatment options are provided. They will mail you information written in layman's terms within twenty-four hours of your call. The staff is personable, very knowledge-able, and helpful. They're grant-funded by the National Cancer Institute. There are two Internet addresses listed above. The first is the general NCI site; the second is a special section I found that provides you detailed information specifically about breast cancer, its causes, and treatments. Their regional office is located at Johns Hopkins. That specific address is below.

CIS Regional Office
Johns Hopkins Oncology Center
550 N. Broadway, Suite 300
Baltimore, MD 21205

American Cancer Society
1599 Clifton Rd. NE
Atlanta, GA 30329
(800) ACS-2345
www.cancer.org

This organization will send information to you on treatment, detection, and prevention as well as provide you connections with your local chapter of the ACS in your immediate area. They also offer three special programs for breast cancer patients.

Pamphlets about breast cancer treatment, causes, the impact the disease has on a woman physically and emotionally, and other information pertinent to women newly diagnosed or facing a recurrence of the disease. These documents are free of charge to callers requesting one copy of the materials.

Reach to Recovery is a program operated by volunteers who have been breast cancer patients themselves. They have completed treatment at least one year ago and attended a special training program designed to teach them how to provide support to women newly diagnosed. Volunteers are "matched" with new patients so that the Reach to Recovery volunteer you speak with is someone who has had the same type of breast cancer as you, similar cultural background, and same treatment. Speaking to someone who's had the same treatment that you are to have can be very helpful. It's ideal to talk with someone who received their treatment at the same institution that you're planning to go to since there are variations in treatments/procedures as I've mentioned before.

CanSurmount and **I Can Cope** are general programs offered by this organization to unite volunteers, patients with cancer (and their families), and health-care professionals in providing educational and emotional support.

Y-ME National Breast Cancer Organization
212 W. Van Buren Street
Chicago, IL 60607
(800) 221-2141
www.Y-ME.org
This is a national organization designed also to provide support to women diagnosed with breast cancer. They also distribute literature about breast cancer treatments. It's staffed by breast cancer survivors who are volunteers. Local chapters also "match" trained breast cancer survivor volunteers with newly diagnosed women seeking support and information as they begin their treatment. The volunteer stays in touch with them throughout their entire treatment program if desired.

National Alliance of Breast Cancer Organizations (NABCO)
9 East 37th Street, 10th floor
New York, NY 10016
(888) 80-NABCO
www.nabco.org
e-mail address: NABCOinfo@aol.com
This is a leading non-profit central resource for information about breast cancer. They provide a network of more than 350 organizations that provide detection, treatment, and care for hundreds of

thousands of women in the U.S. Their website provides current information about breast cancer, updates on breast-related events and activities, and links to other breast cancer websites. They post information about clinical research trials. They have a "resource router," list national support groups, and conduct surveys on-line as well.

The Susan G. Komen Foundation
Occidental Tower
5005 LBJ Freeway, Suite 250
Dallas, TX 75244
(800) IM-AWARE
www.komen.org

This is a national volunteer organization seeking to eradicate breast cancer as a life-threatening disease, working through local chapters and the Race for the Cure events in more than sixty cities. The Foundation is the largest private funder of breast cancer research in the United States. The Komen Alliance is a comprehensive program for the research, education, diagnosis, and treatment of breast disease.

National Breast Cancer Coalition (NBCC)
1701 L Street NW
Washington, DC 20036
(800) 622-2838
www.natlbcc.org

Formed in 1991 with more than 140 organizations representing several million patients, professionals, women, and their families and friends, NBCC has a significant impact on general awareness about breast cancer. They also have a major influence on public policy.

The Wellness Community
2716 Ocean Park Boulevard, Suite 1040
Santa Monica, CA 90405
(310) 314-2555
e-mail address: TWCNATL@aol.com
This program has extensive support and education programs
which encourage emotional recovery and a feeling of wellness for
people battling all types of cancer. All services are free. Their head-
quarters address is listed above but there might be a local chapter
in your immediate area now. With breast cancer affecting more
than 180,000 women each year, the Wellness Community has taken
the time to develop special programs exclusively for women with
breast cancer.

Mothers Supporting Daughters with Breast Cancer (MSDBC)
C/O Charmayne Dierker
21710 Bayshore Road
Chestertown, MD 21620-4401
(410) 778-1982
www.mothersdaughters.com
This national non-profit organization was founded in March,
1995. It's designed to provide educational information about breast
cancer treatment and emotional support to mothers who have
daughters battling breast cancer. The program connects a mother
with a mother volunteer who has already had a daughter diagnosed
with breast cancer and treated. The volunteer provides the mother
emotional support and guidance on how to be more helpful to her
daughter from point of diagnosis through to completion of treatment. The organization also has a "Mother's Handbook" and
"Daughter's Companion Booklet" which provide some constructive suggestions how a mother can be helpful to her daughter
during such a medical crisis. All materials are provided free of
charge. The organization was created in recognition that a mother
feels helpless when she learns that her daughter has breast cancer.
A woman needs as much support as she can get when she learns she

has breast cancer, including support from her mother. Her mother may be too distressed to provide constructive support, however, which can negatively affect her daughter. This program provides the needed support to assist the mother to be able to cope herself and in turn provide support to her daughter. A mother doesn't necessarily have to be a biological mother either—any woman who is fulfilling such a support role qualifies.

The National Coalition for Cancer Survivorship (NCCS)
1010 Wayne Avenue, 5th floor
Silver Spring, MD 20910
(301) 650-8868
www.cansearch.org

This organization raises awareness of cancer survivorship through its publications, quarterly newsletters, and education. The organization seeks to eliminate the stigma of cancer and provides advocacy for insurance, employment, and legal rights for people with cancer. NCCS facilitates networking among cancer organizations, serves as an information clearinghouse and encourages the study of cancer survivorship. On the national level, they provide public policy leadership on legislation, regulatory, and financial matters and promote responsible advocacy among national organizations.

Yellow Pages

Local chapter of the American Cancer Society—Use the ACS to receive literature about breast cancer support groups in your area.

Mastectomy Supply Stores—Sometimes these stores have sales on mastectomy bras! It's smart to call them around Memorial Day and Labor Day for the best buys on mastectomy swimwear, too.

Wig Stores—If you're anticipating chemotherapy and the drugs used usually cause hair loss, it's recommended that you're fitted for a wig before you start your therapy. These stores often carry pamphlets on creative ways to wear scarves on your head as well.

Land's End, Inc.
1 Land's End Lane
Dodgeville, WI 53595
(800) 356-4444
This company carries mastectomy bathing suits as well as tank tops that are cut closer than most around the arm hole area—perfect for women who have had the axillary node dissections. The bathing suits are frequently on sale, too. Worth checking out!

B & B Breast Prosthesis Company
P.O. Box 5731
2417 Bank Drive, Suite 201
Boise, ID 83705
(800) 343-9696
They make a special breast prosthesis, designed by a breast cancer survivor, which serves as an alternative to heavier silicone breast forms. It fits in a regular bra and is made of nylon and cotton cushioned with fiberfill. It's washable and costs around $70, including shipping.

Jodee Bra Inc.
3100 N. 20th Avenue
Hollywood, FL 33020
(800) 865-6333
Louis Rose, vice president of Jodee and a national consultant says, "Every woman needs to know what to look for in a good fitting, for she fits herself everyday. When she goes to a store to be fitted, she should have the following check points to assure a good fitting, because not all fitters are equal in their training and experience."
The checkpoints that are recommended are listed below.
1. Does your bra touch the center breastbone? Good separation prevents "peekout."
2. Does your bra ride up? Wear it snug, not loose, so the bandeau can work.

3. Does your breast form (prosthesis) feel heavy? Adjust the straps so the breast form is close to your body.

4. Does the breast form projection match your natural size? Try smaller or larger breast forms.

5. Are you wearing straps close to your neck to prevent grabbing and creating tilted shoulders? (A common cause of shoulder and neck pain).

6. Is there a depressed area above the breast form? Sew in a foam tab to fill this cavity. (These tabs are available in the Jodee catalog. I haven't seen them available elsewhere.)

7. Does your bra pull or twist to the side? Reasons for this can be:

    a) Cup form too small on natural size.

    b) Breast form too light in weight.

    c) Flesh from underarm causes bra to twist or slide.

Use foam cushion to fill in this area. (These cushions are very hard to find but are available through Jodee.)

The Johns Hopkins Breast Center
601 N. Caroline Street
Balitimore, MD 21287
(410) 955-4851
www.med.jhu.edu/breastcenter

If you want to receive care or desire a second opinion, this is an excellent facility, complete with top-notch health-care providers recognized nationally and internationally for their expertise in the field. The Breast Center has a website that offers a great deal of information for women and their families in need of breast cancer information. The Breast Cancer Patient's Bill of Rights is available on the home page and was written by a team of breast cancer survivor volunteers who work at the Breast Center with me. You will also find Artemis, our electronic medical journal, that provides you with a monthly update of the latest information regarding breast cancer research and treatment—and you can subscribe to it free. There's also a great deal of educational information about breast cancer and its treatment—one of the reasons why this website has received national awards in excellence for patient education information. My work e-mail address is also available at this site if you need to reach me in a professional capacity.

The Breast Center strives to meet not only the physical needs of a woman, but also the emotional needs of a patient, and those who are supporting her at home. The patient education program is outstanding. The faculty—all of whom are oncologists with breast cancer expertise in surgery, medical oncology, radiation oncology, and radiology—are excellent. This has been confirmed with the results of the patient satisfaction/quality-of-care surveys we conduct with our patients. We invited women, no matter where they received their treatment, to go to our website and complete the satisfaction survey themselves. It's connected to a database for the purpose of producing reports that lets us benchmark with other facilities. Our long-range goal is to develop national quality standards for breast cancer diagnosis and treatment so that women, no matter where they get treated, can feel assured that they're in the very best of hands.

Patients treated at Johns Hopkins are given the option to be "matched" with a Johns Hopkins Breast Cancer Survivor Volunteer who is the same age, stage of disease, and has already completed the treatment plan the patient is about to embark upon. The survivor volunteer provides support all the way through to the completion of treatment, if the patient desires. This program, which I developed in 1997, is the only one of its kind and we hope other hospitals adopt a similar model and provide this level of support in the future, too.

If you come to the Johns Hopkins Breast Center, let me know! I'll do my best to meet you at the time of your visit. If you're faced with the challenge of becoming a new "club member," I want to be of personal assistance to you and your family as you go through the steps necessary in the transformation from a victim to a survivor of breast cancer.

OncoLink
University of Pennsylvania Cancer Center's website
www.OncoLink.org

OncoLink was the very first multimedia oncology information resource on the Internet and remains a good source for cancer information, including breast cancer. There are several videos available from that website that provide educational information and support worth checking out as well.

Intelihealth
www.intelihealth.com

This is an excellent website for medical information of all types, including breast cancer. The "breast cancer zone" information is exclusively provided by Hopkins faculty. Information is updated weekly, so visit it often!

Survivors' Club
www.survivorsclub.org

Survivors' Club is a website that offers cancer patients and their families hope, support, and online friendship. This site is unique from any other breast site that I've seen. Breast cancer patients voluntarily enter their own stories into an online database. Any breast cancer patient can search and find others that have a similar "profile" to their own. For example, one could find another forty-three-year-old woman with DCIS of the right breast who lives in California. Patients with similar profiles are free to provide each other support, comfort, and friendship via e-mail, private chat rooms, and message boards!

If you want to be prayed for by others, you can add your name (or a loved one's name) to a prayer list that's widely distributed. Interviews with leading cancer experts on hot topics appear regularly along with selected articles on breast cancer research. Online conferences feature celebrity guests. Important issues, like the establishment of a national standard of care, are followed. Another unique feature is that family members of survivors and/or lost loved ones can post messages of support and cherished pictures.

Appendix C

QUESTIONS WOMEN WITH BREAST CANCER FREQUENTLY ASK ABOUT HEALTH INSURANCE BENEFITS

From my past experience, as well as from my conversations with many breast cancer patients, there are some key questions that arise related to health insurance coverage that might be helpful for you to know. Concerns about what your health insurance does and doesn't cover can add unnecessary anxiety and worry to you at a time that you don't need it. By being proactive, you can contact your insurance company and get information up front about what they do and don't cover. This information below will also help advise you how to optimize the coverage you do have.

Will my insurance company cover my mastectomy/lumpectomy surgery if I'm an inpatient?

Most insurance companies, including managed-care organizations, will cover an overnight stay. However, there has been a trend toward outpatient surgery unless you're having reconstruction done at the same time or you have other medical conditions warranting hospitalization. Depending on where you live, there might be specific legislation relating to ensuring coverage for overnight stays as well. The need to be an inpatient or an ambulatory surgery patient should be decided by you with input from your surgeon. Discuss this with your surgeon first, then talk with your insurance company if you're planning to be hospitalized. Johns Hopkins makes it the patient's choice to be an inpatient or outpatient for mastectomy surgery without reconstruction based on input from her surgeon. We are strong believers that only hospitals who have developed comprehensive patient education programs which are conducted in advance of the patient's surgery should be performing mastectomies on an outpatient basis. We know from experience, however, that patients prefer going home the day of surgery 93 percent of the time and do very well. They score us high on patient satisfaction surveys and feel confident that they made the right choice in electing to have their surgery performed on an outpatient basis. It requires a commitment of time, effort, and resources to develop a program that works well, however. Unfortunately, not many facilities have invested this time and energy. So ask your doctor how many patients have been done on an outpatient basis if he/she is recommending that you have your surgery done in this way. Pressure from insurance carriers shouldn't dictate whether you're treated on an inpatient or outpatient basis. Decisions about this must rest with you and your doctor.

I don't know if I want to have reconstruction done yet. Will it still be covered if I choose to wait until a later time, or is it only covered if done as part of my breast cancer surgery now? Will my insurance cover any type of reconstruction, such as tram flap, saline implant, or dorsal flap?

Most insurance companies will cover reconstruction of all types, but check to see if they place a time limit when you can have it done. This was legislation passed in December, 1997, requiring that all insurance companies cover reconstruction of all types for an unlimited length of time after the initial mastectomy surgery. Presently, there are some insurance companies who require that the reconstruction be done within one year of the initial mastectomy surgery, if it's to be a covered benefit.

I've decided not to have reconstruction. I'd prefer to wear a breast prosthesis. How expensive are they, and how much will my insurance cover?

This is a tricky question. Breast prostheses range in price from

$50 (made of cloth with tiny pillows for fillers inside) to $1,400 (made of silicone and created from a mold of the other breast), with the standard prosthesis costing about $350. Silicone prostheses usually come with a two-year warranty. There are also breast prostheses designed for swimming; these range in price from $15 to $40. If an insurance company only covers one prosthesis, make sure you submit the sales receipt of the permanent silicone breast prosthesis to your insurance company, not the receipt of the swimmer's prosthesis or a less-expensive model such as the cloth prosthesis. Since the insurance company will only cover one, you need to submit the more expensive one to them, otherwise you'll be stuck with a large bill and they will have technically paid for a prosthesis, even if it's a swimmer's model or cloth model. This can result in a serious financial hardship, which is avoidable if you know how to submit your insurance bills up front. Also, make sure you get a prescription from your surgeon ordering that you be fitted for a breast prosthesis as well as a mastectomy bra. Without the prescription, you'll probably have trouble getting fitted and will definitely have trouble getting your insurance company to pay the bill. Most insurance companies pay 80 to 100 percent of the bill for prostheses. Some companies are rigid and only cover the purchase of one prosthesis for a lifetime. This is an important benefit to ask about. Other companies will cover reimbursement for a prosthesis every two years.

What happens if my body changes in size and my prosthesis no longer fits properly? Can I get a replacement, and is it covered by my insurance?

Most insurance companies will cover replacements for this reason, provided there's a prescription from your doctor stating the reason for the replacement.

Can I go anywhere to get a breast prosthesis, or are there only certain locations approved for me to go?

Most insurance companies will let a patient go anywhere she

chooses. It's wise to choose a store that employs certified fitters who are specially trained to fit women for breast prostheses. Being fitted for a mastectomy bra and/or prosthesis is very intimidating, and can be degrading if not done by a highly professional staff dedicated to making the experience a nonstressful one. Ask the health-care professionals if they have a list of stores they recommend who employ certified fitters. You'll probably find that many of the mastectomy supply shops are owned by women who have had breast cancer themselves. These women have chosen to help others like you and me—they know how you feel because they've been there themselves. Feel free to ask when you call to make a fitting appointment if any of the fitters are breast cancer survivors.

Are mastectomy bras covered by my insurance, and if so, how many will they cover per year?

There is some variance among insurance companies about this particular benefit. Most insurers will cover two bras per year, provided they're accompanied with a prescription from a doctor. During October, National Breast Cancer Awareness Month, many mastectomy supply shops have sales on their mastectomy supply items. This is especially important if your insurance company doesn't cover reimbursement for mastectomy bras beyond the initial coverage of two bras. Bras are expensive—take advantage of sales! (Mastectomy bathing suits, by the way, aren't covered by insurance companies. These items are almost always on sale around Labor Day.)

I've been told that I might need chemotherapy. Is it covered by my insurance? What if I choose to participate in a clinical trial? What drugs aren't covered?

This varies from company to company. Call and ask them specific questions. It's best to also ask the oncologist if a research grant will cover any drug and treatment costs if you do participate in a clinical trial. There is a positive trend developing now, which is good news, of insurance companies covering health expenses related to clinical trial participation.

I might need radiation therapy. Is this covered by my insurance?

Check to see what sites are covered for radiation therapy. Sometimes patients assume they will receive all medical care at the place they were diagnosed and initially treated, and are later surprised to discover that the site for radiation treatment is in a different location and will be provided by health care professionals who aren't part of the patient's original treatment team. If this is the case, you need to know up front to prevent anxiety about it later.

Based on my understanding of the type of chemotherapy I'll be receiving, I might lose my hair. Will my insurance company cover the cost of a wig? How soon can I get one? Does my hair have to be completely gone in order to get one?

Many companies do cover this expense. However, it might require sending a letter to the insurance company from your doctor. If they don't cover it, check with the American Cancer Society or with the Breast Center where you're being treated; they might have access to wigs for you if this is a financial burden for you. There are various organizations and hospitals that have a supply for "recycling" to newly diagnosed patients who are in need of such an item. It's advisable to be fitted for a wig before you begin to lose your hair. This way, the wig will be easily matched to your hair color and hairstyle.

I've been told that I may need a bone marrow transplant as part of my chemotherapy treatment. Is this covered by my insurance?

This is an expensive procedure, which needs more research to determine if it's helping women beat this disease. Your insurance company may cover part of it or possibly all of it. There's wide variation among insurance carriers about this. Some companies still consider its value as experimental and therefore don't cover it at all. If you're anticipating needing this procedure, check with your insurance company and get information in writing from them about what they do and don't cover relating to this specific treatment.

My doctor plans to do my procedure (mastectomy or lumpectomy with axillary node removal) as an outpatient procedure. Arrangements are going to be made by the Breast Center for a home health nurse to come to my home the night of my surgery and the next day. Is this expense covered by my insurance?

Most insurance companies do cover home health care following this type of surgery. They usually cover two visits and there must be extenuating medical circumstances to warrant approval of additional visits. There are special forms that the doctor or nurse fills out for the insurance company and for the home health nurse to assist with ensuring coverage. Insurance companies usually contract with specific home health care agencies, too. Ideally, the home health nurse caring for you is familiar with outpatient mastectomy care. (Johns Hopkins has trained home health-care nurses specifically for this purpose to ensure they know what's expected of them when conducting a home-health visit. This better ensures continuity of care for you.)

I might be switching insurance companies in the middle of my treatment. Will my new insurance company cover the continuation of my current cancer treatments?

If at all possible, it's best not to switch insurance companies in the midst of treatment. There can be serious problems with insurance coverage for the continuation of your breast cancer care. If you're leaving your present place of employment, you might want to strongly consider continuing your current insurance coverage by paying the monthly premiums yourself at least until your treatments are completed. You should also check with your new insurance company about their policies regarding "pre-existing conditions." Some companies picking you up as a new member will continue your coverage for breast cancer treatment and others may not for a specified period of time.

What can I do to influence changes in my insurance coverage if I think that my insurance company is being unreasonable about my treatment benefits?

First, talk with the member relations manager for your insurance company to see if you can come to some agreement about what's reasonable coverage and what's not. If you're unsuccessful in getting satisfactory help, you may need your doctor to write a letter on your behalf explaining the medical need for certain treatments and such. If the problem is one related to your insurance company not providing a specific benefit at all or a limited benefit (for example, one prosthesis for a lifetime), you may want to write to your insurance commissioner or even contact your local Congressman or Senator who may be able to promote legislation requiring certain types of coverage for all women unrelated to the type of insurance they have.

Lillie Shockney is a national speaker and published author on breast cancer and the director of education and outreach at Johns Hopkins Breast Center. A breast cancer survivor herself, she is also a registered nurse who holds a bachelor's degree in health- 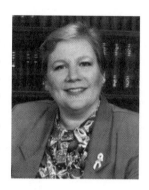 care administration and a master's degree in administrative science from Johns Hopkins University. She is the recipient of numerous awards including Intel's Internet health hero; *Shape* magazine and the National Race for the Cure's "Circle of Life" Award. She and her mother, Charmayne Dierker, formed Mothers Supporting Daughters with Breast Cancer to help mothers and daughters cope with the stresses of a cancer diagnosis. In 1999, the American Cancer Society chose Shockney as its "Voice of Hope." More recently, Upjohn & Pharmacia selected her as one of their "Unsung Heroes of Breast Cancer."